Atlas of
HUMAN HISTOLOGY
AND ULTRASTRUCTURE

Atlas of
HUMAN HISTOLOGY
AND ULTRASTRUCTURE

J. L. MATTHEWS, Ph.D.

*Professor and Chairman, Department of Anatomy
Baylor University Graduate Division and Dental
College, Dallas, Texas*

and

J. H. MARTIN, Ph.D.

*Department of Anatomy and Department of Pathology
Baylor University Medical Center, Dallas, Texas*

1971

LEA & FEBIGER   PHILADELPHIA

ISBN 0-8121-0347-5

Published in Great Britain by Henry Kimpton Publishers
Library of Congress Catalog Card Number: 72–157470
Printed in the United States of America

FOREWORD

THE advances in the study of cellular fine structure in the past thirty years are astonishing. The electron microscope has, indeed, proved a tool of many disciplines from metallurgy to pure biological science, but perhaps it has served most significantly by bringing the disciplines of biological chemistry and morphology under one roof. Indeed, pure biological science currently is advancing primarily through the contributions of the structural and chemical disciplines interpretable as cell physiology.

Rudolph Virchow succeeded in centering the attention of investigators on the cell as the unit of life and also as the ultimate seat of diseases manifested by altered function. The problem in the late nineteenth century was, however, that reliable normal tissue histology had to be learned before pathological histology could be developed as a useful tool. The same can be said for ultrastructural morphology in the twentieth century.

The present contribution by Matthews and Martin one hundred years after Virchow advances the state of our knowledge of ultrastructure of the cell by satisfying a need. As pointed out by Keith Porter and Mary Bonneville, Johannes Rhodin, Don Fawcett and others, there is an urgent need for base-line comparative information on fine structure, specifically in the human. Many of the electron photomicrographs in prior atlases came from laboratory animals and, indeed, in many cases animal tissues were the only comparable base-line fine structure for comparison with human tissues. In this work all tissues are human, and the atlas will give all investigators an additional sense of security in the interpretation of fine structure. In addition, the comparison of thin section and light microscopy to human electron microscopy is most illuminating.

GEORGE J. RACE, M.D., Ph.D.
Pathologist-in-Chief
Baylor University Medical Center
Dallas, Texas

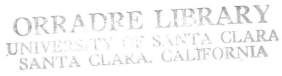
v

PREFACE

With the new techniques and the constantly increasing knowledge in the field of microscopic anatomy, the student faces a continuous task in keeping up with the influx of new material. This requires surveillance of the widely dispersed sources of microscopic and especially ultrastructural anatomy in the literature. This volume was prepared in an attempt partially to alleviate this problem.

An effort has been made to produce an atlas useful both to beginning students in histology and to practicing professional microscopists, anatomists, physiologists and pathologists. To achieve this objective, human tissues were used exclusively. Recent literature references are included for further information on the subjects presented.

The transition from the viewing of conventional preparations of tissues embedded in paraffin cut at 3 to 7 microns to the viewing of tissues at the electron-microscope level has been a major obstacle to orientation. To facilitate this transition, stains effective on tissues embedded in plastic and having the character of the routine H & E are used in this atlas. Thin plastic sections (0.5 microns) provide several advantages. The optimal limit of resolution of the light microscope (0.2 microns) is realized. Preservation of cytologic detail is enhanced by the primary aldehyde fixation, postosmication, and the elimination of the need for removal of the embedding media. Reduction of several solvent stages in the preparation of tissues for thin sections further reduces the leeching out of many cellular components. Intensity of contrast has been increased over prior phase-optical preparations using monochromatic stains, but only recently has color contrast been practicable. The thin sections in this atlas were stained with a polychrome stain closely approximating the H & E differentiation familiar to most microscopists. Photomicrographs of H & E stained sections, polychrome stained thin plastic sections, "adjacent" sections, and electron micrographs of these tissues are presented sequentially in an effort to correlate microscopic structure and ultrastructure.

Specimens for this atlas were obtained from biopsy specimens, areas peripheral to surgical pathology specimens, and, in rare instances, from autopsy specimens. Several plates include electron micrographs of human tissues not previously available. It is hoped that the combination of photomicrographs and electron micrographs will provide a basis for furthering an understanding of both normal and diseased tissues.

The authors wish to thank the following people for their contributions in the acquisition of tissues for this atlas: Doctors W. B. Kingsley, R. N. Walter, F. G. Spruill, J. B. Belue, C. J. Helling, A. L. Raines, V. H. Lary, R. G. Chambers, J. H. Coenhour, M. Gilbert, D. S. Branch and D. Vendrell.

Technical assistance was rendered by J. Willis, J. Roan, J. Fenter, A. Barnett, E. Kirklin, G. Vineyard, A. Fields, S. Bennett, H. Shaw, H. Hitchcock, and graduate students F. Carson, H. W. Sampson, W. L. Davis, T. E. Croley, D. L. Murphey, J. E. Aschenbrenner and B. E. Avery.

Special appreciation is extended to Miss Freida Carson who produced several of the blood and marrow cell micrographs and who was responsible for organizing the collection of tissues in her capacity as chief technician of the Department of Surgical Pathology; to Dr. J. A. Lynn who helped to organize the atlas; to Dr. G. J. Race for making facilities and equipment available and for his encouragement and support; to Dr. R. E. Dill for reviewing the manuscript; and to Mrs. Joan Nash for her secretarial contributions.

J. L. MATTHEWS
Dallas, Texas   J. H. MARTIN

CONTENTS

The Cell

Plate 1 — CELL

Figure 1. Electron micrograph of secretory cell of gastric glands. The cells in this figure were selected to depict several of the cellular components to be discussed in the succeeding plates. Cells vary in size, shape and content. Intracellular components and their distribution often reflect the special activities of these units. The nucleus (N) contains a nucleolus (Nu) and shows clumping of the granular chromatin, particularly adjacent to the nuclear membrane (NM). The nonclumped euchromatin is the site of genetic determination of cell morphology and function. Nuclear pores (NP) are seen in the nuclear membrane. The cytoplasm contains mitochondria (M) essential for the production of energy-rich compounds via oxygen utilization. Rough-surfaced membranes of endoplasmic reticulum (ER) ramify throughout the cell and serve as sites of protein synthesis at the ribosomes, the small granules giving the membranes their rough appearance. Ribosomes also occur free in the cytoplasm. A Golgi complex (G) consisting of flattened sacs and vesicles is interposed between secretion granules (SG), a product invested in membrane at the Golgi complex and secreted at the cell's free surface. Other organelles such as lysosomes and centrioles, and inclusions such as glycogen, pigment, etc., are not seen in this section. Electron microscopy requires that the section being viewed be very thin so that electrons can be transmitted through the cell. Hence, the same cell is cut several times in succeeding sections with the microtome and only a small part of the total cell content is included in any micrograph. The plasma membrane of these cells touches a basal lamina (BL) which is the beginning of an area of connective tissue. The plasma membrane (PM) is not straight; rather, interdigitations of adjacent cells may be seen at the arrow. These membranes are separated by at least 20 mμ. The free surfaces of cells may contain phagocytic or pinocytotic vesicles and projections in the form of microvilli. Motile structures in the form of cilia or flagella may be present. The plasma membrane is the special interface between the cell content and the environment; it thus has several features relative to permeability, dielectric properties, and systems for active and passive transport. It is a trilaminar structure consisting of two outer dense lines separated by a less dense area.

Cells and cell products serving a specific function comprise tissues, while tissues organized for a common function constitute organs; organs serving specific functions are the basis of systems. Hence, the cell is the fundamental unit of an organism. ($\times$14,700)

2

PLATE 1

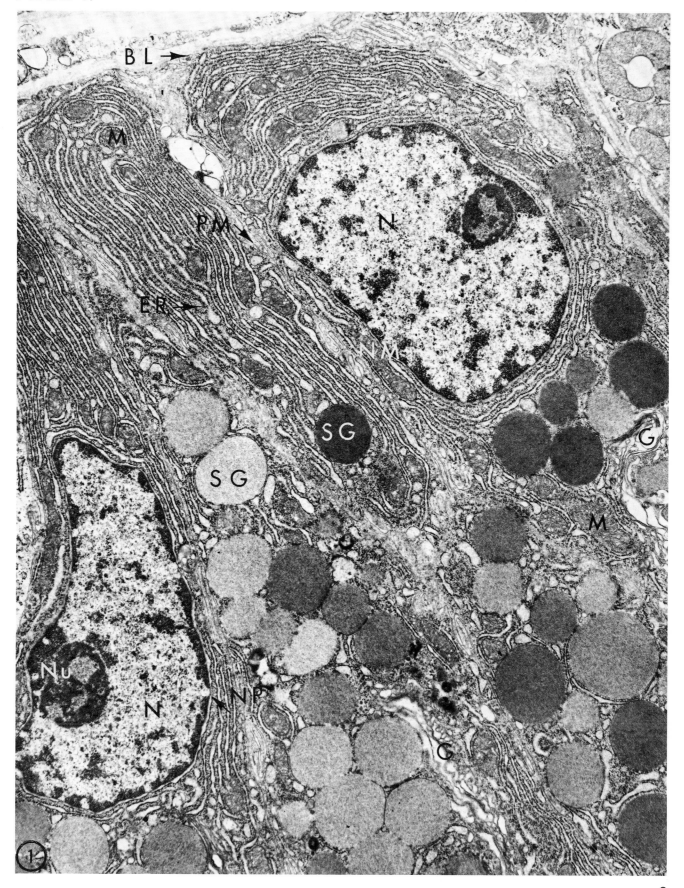

Plate 2 – MITOCHONDRIA

Figure 1. Electron micrograph of cross section of skeletal muscle. In this figure, the mitochondria are elongated branched sacs occupying the sarcoplasm between myofibrils. They are also in immediate proximity to a lipid (Li) droplet, a common relationship seen in many cell types. The mitochondria have a double-membrane arrangement. The inner membrane is infolded to form the cristae mitochondriales (Cr). Mitochondria contain all of the enzymes of the Krebs cycle, and all of the enzymes required for coupled phosphorylation and fatty-acid oxidation. They are prime users of oxygen, and have been called the "power house" of the cell because of their production of adenosine triphosphate (ATP). ($\times$36,000)

Figure 2. Electron micrograph of leukocyte mitochondria. These mitochondria (M) have a tubular profile in longitudinal section and a round profile in cross section. Mitochondria may attain 10 μ in length to 5 μ in diameter, but are usually smaller. They are well within the resolving capacity of the light microscope. Mitochondria readily change shape and size. This mitochondrion contains an electron-dense granule (MG). Analysis of these granules has shown that some of them are soluble in lipid solvents while others persist following extraction and microincineration, indicating a high mineral content. These granules contain calcium, magnesium, phosphate and a protein in bone and cartilage cells. ($\times$55,000)

Figure 3. Electron micrograph of salivary duct cell. The numbers of mitochondria (M) in this cell are enormous and each mitochondrion is filled with cristae. Both the number and size of mitochondria can vary in cells. Cells with large numbers of mitochondria are presumed to be active in some energy-requiring activity, such as secretion, contraction, etc. General cells have 200 to 400 mitochondria; they may, however, have very few, as in the lymphocyte, or more than 2500. This view is of one very thin section. A count of all the mitochondria of this cell sectioned serially would be enormous. The nucleus (N) and plasma membrane (PM) are indicated. ($\times$15,000)

Figure 4. Electron micrograph of mitochondria of secreting cell. In this view, the continuity of the inner mitochondrial membrane can be followed into the interior as it forms the cristae (Cr) membranes. Each of the membranes appears as a trilaminar unit membrane. The space between the two unit membranes is about 10 mμ. High resolution microscopy of negatively stained cristae has shown them to have small 10-mμ knobs evenly spaced along the membrane. The knobs are attached to the cristae membranes by narrow stalks. The precise localization of all mitochondrial enzymes is not yet resolved, but some enzymes appear to reside on these knobs while others occupy the matrix between cristae. ($\times$57,600)

4

PLATE 2

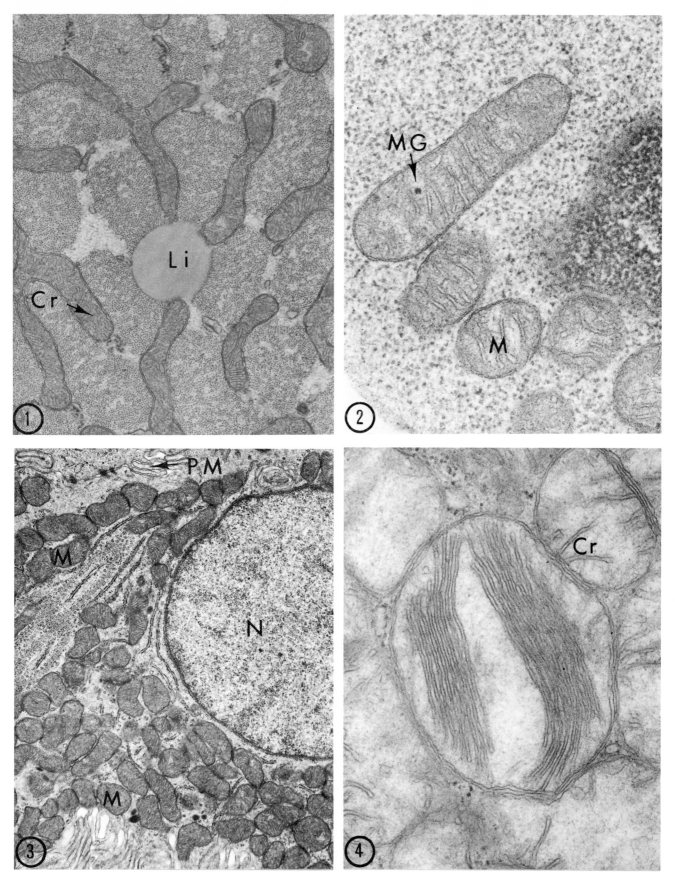

Plate 3 — LYSOSOMES

Figure 1. Electron micrograph of Kupffer cell. The sinusoidal spaces (S) of the liver are lined with phagocytic Kupffer cells (KC) separated from the liver parenchyma cells (PC) by a narrow space, the space of Disse (SD). Microvilli (Mv) from both cell types project into the space. Several organelles limited by a single membrane, the lysosomes (Ly), appear as rounded bodies of varying size. These lysosomes contain electron-dense granules, lipid droplets, and myelin figures but do not have the highly organized internal structure of the mitochondria. The lysosome contains digestive enzymes capable of reducing large molecules to simpler constituents which can be used by mitochondrial enzymes. These structures are particularly rich in acid phosphatases and hydrolases and can be identified histochemically by the Gomori method. ($\times$8,000)

Figure 2. Electron micrograph of reticular cell in the spleen. This cell contains a nucleus (N) in which the dispersed (euchromatin) and condensed (heterochromatin) chromatin are readily delineated. Free ribosomes (Ri), rough-surfaced endoplasmic reticulum (ER) and a mitochondrion (M) are seen in the cytoplasm. Lysosomes (Ly) containing a dense matrix and irregular dense inclusions are randomly distributed. Inspection of the mitochondrial membrane reveals a double-membrane structure with the inner membrane projecting inward forming the cristae. The lysosome is bounded by a single membrane. Erythrocytes (RBC) occupy the sinusoidal spaces between reticular cells. The reticular cells rest upon an incomplete basal lamina (BL). ($\times$7,500)

Figure 3. Electron micrograph of a macrophage in marrow tissue. In this figure, a large macrophage (Mp) has completely encompassed a neutrophil (Ne) with a several-lobed nucleus, indicative of an old leukocyte. A cytoplasmic process (P) of the macrophage extends beyond the neutrophil, which is surrounded on all sides by a thin layer of macrophage cytoplasm. Several electron-dense lysosomes (Ly) are situated at the neutrophil surface. Other lysosomes of varying sizes occupy other parts of the cytoplasm. Substances acted on by lysosomes may arise exogenously by heterophagy as seen here, or endogenously by autophagy. Some of the hydrolytic products of their action may be excreted by the cell, a process called exocytosis. These vesicles are called residual bodies (RB) before extrusion and often contain lipids in various forms. In autophagic processes, parts of cell organelles may be recognized within the autophagic vacuole or cytolysosome. An erythrocyte (E) and other leukocytes surround the macrophage. ($\times$9,500)

PLATE 3

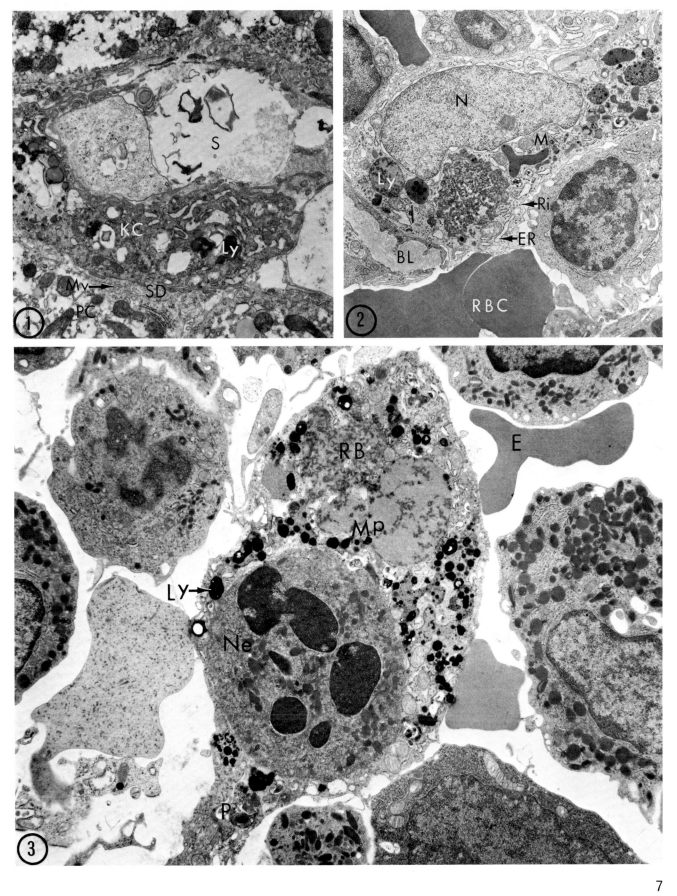

Plate 4 — GOLGI COMPLEX

Figure 1. Electron micrograph of Golgi complex of an immature eosinophil. The Golgi complex (G) is close to the nucleus (N) and surrounds a centriole (Ce). Specific granules (SG) of the eosinophil are seen in varying stages of maturation. The ultrastructure shows a series of nongranular membranes arranged in parallel sheets with one end closed, producing an internal cisterna. This may be likened to a single sheet of paper folded upon itself, producing a closed end with a related cisterna. Several folded papers arranged in a stack or tube would serve as a model for this complex. Often a stack of Golgi vesicles shows some curvature, producing a convex (formative) and a concave (mature or secretory) face. These cisternal structures vary in length. The cisternal space measures about 15 nm across. ($\times$22,000)

Figure 2. Electron micrograph of a cell containing a small, relatively inactive Golgi complex (G). The lamellae of this complex may be compared with the rough-surfaced endoplasmic reticulum (ER) in this view. ($\times$12,300)

Figure 3. Electron micrograph of Golgi complex (G) in a monocyte. The Golgi complex usually occupies a juxtanuclear position, and is often found within an indented area of the nucleus (N) approaching the cell center, a region also occupied by centrioles (Ce). With phase microscopy, this region of cytoplasm might have a refractive index different from that of the surrounding cytoplasm. The Golgi complex in this view shows the characteristic curvature of the Golgi lamellae. The convex (formative) face is indicated by the arrow. Small vesicles are immediately adjacent to the cisternal units, particularly at the formative face. Larger vesicles are seen at one end and along the opposite surface (the mature face) of the units. These large vesicles contain material of various densities, and have been shown to represent secretion vesicles in different states of maturity. Proteins are believed to be brought to these cisternae via membranes of the endoplasmic reticulum. These proteins and other materials are ultimately condensed within the closed end of the cisterna. Budding and enlargement of this end and budding of the mature face represent the formative steps in production of secretion granules. ($\times$15,700)

Figure 4. Electron micrograph of mucus-secreting cell. The Golgi complex (G) is usually close to the nucleus and is found on the lumen (L) side of a secretory exocrine cell. The size of this complex varies with secretory activity. Although proteins are brought to the Golgi complex, experiments with isotopic precursors indicate that some polysaccharides may arise in these structures *de novo*. It is difficult clearly to define the outer limits of the Golgi complex because of the migration of large secretion vesicles (SV) from the complex and because of the distribution of smooth- and rough-surfaced endoplasmic reticulum (ER). One prime function of this complex appears to be the investing of secretory products within limiting membranes; however, numerous nonsecretory cells have distinct Golgi complexes. The membrane-invested secretion granules fill the apex of the cell, and some are fused with the plasma membrane (PM). ($\times$18,900)

PLATE 11

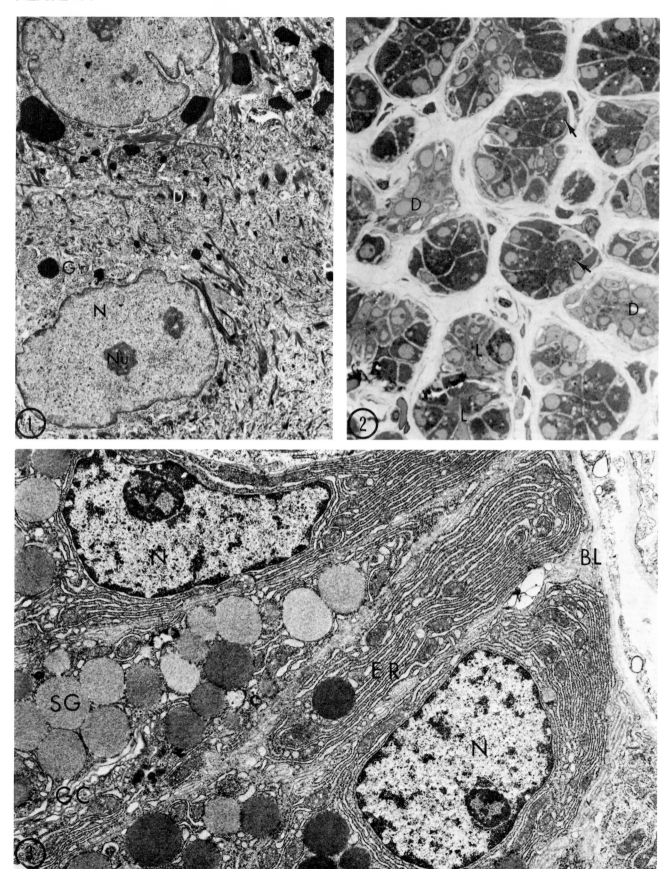

Plate 12 – CELL INCLUSIONS: PIGMENTS

Figure 1.   Electron micrograph of lipofuscin granules. Pigments in tissues may be classi-fied as endogenous or exogenous. Exogenous pigments may originate from foods, as in the case with carotenoids, or from metals such as lead and silver, or they may gain entrance through the respiratory passages in the form of coal tars, etc.

Endogenous pigments may be synthesized within cells or they may arise from degradation of materials within the body such as hemoglobin. Lipofuscin granules (LG) are irregularly shaped, membrane-bound endogenous structures with an amorphous matrix in which electron-dense particles and occasional myelin figures may be found. Forming lipofuscin granules may have an internal lamellar structure, as in the granule (ILG) at the top. These structures increase in number with age and are most abundant in liver, neurons, and cardiac muscle. Lipofuscin granules have some esterase and hydrolase activity and may represent degradative products of lysosomal activity. In light microscopy, they are yellow brown. In cardiac muscle, shown here, the granules first form adjacent to the nucleus and extend into the cytoplasm between mitochondria (M) and myofibrils. A portion of an intercalated disc is seen at the upper left. (×25,000)

Figure 2.   Electron micrograph of melanocyte. Melanin granules (Gr) are special products of melanocytes. These granules are intensely osmophilic and appear homoge-neous in the mature state. Melanin granules are limited by a single membrane and form in the Golgi complex. Vesicles forming in the Golgi complex accu-mulate a protein with the tyrosinase activity essential for the formation of melanin. Forming melanin granules are called melanosomes (Me). The limiting membrane is readily viewed in these structures, as are internal protein lamellae having a beaded or cross-striated appearance. These strands are believed to contain the tyrosinase-rich protein. The lamellar appearance of the melano-somes is ultimately obscured as increasing amounts of melanin are deposited within the melanosome. Recent reports indicate that melanin granule shapes may be a function of race. (×40,700)

Figure 3.   Electron micrograph of melanosome. A limiting membrane (L) of a melano-some surrounds clusters of protein lamellae (LP) having a beaded appearance. Increasing deposits of melanin will obscure the lamellar pattern. (×66,500)

PLATE 12

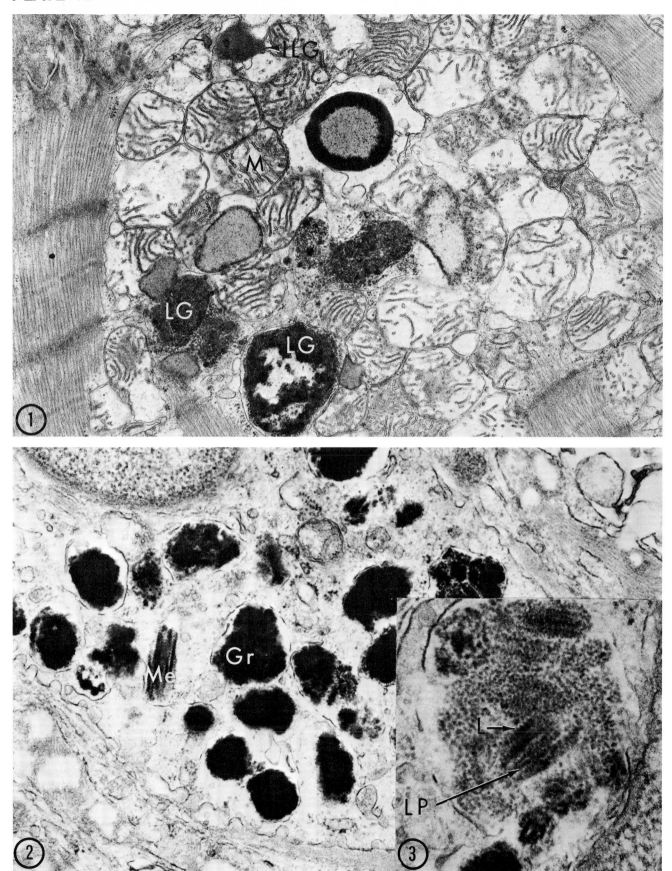

Plate 13 — CELL DIVISION

Figure 1.   Photomicrograph of squash preparation of metaphase chromosomes. The normal diploid chromosome number in man is 46. This complement of chromosomes is most readily seen when colchicine is given to an animal or, in this case, is added to a cell culture in which cell division is occurring. Colchicine temporarily arrests the mitotic process at metaphase, a feature useful for accumulating larger numbers of cells in this division stage.

   The cells were not sectioned in this preparation, but were spread on a glass slide and stained with Feulgen stain, which gives a positive reaction with DNA, a major chromosome constituent. The nuclear membrane, plasma membrane, nucleolus, organelles, etc. contain little or no DNA and thus did not stain. Each metaphase chromosome (Ch) consists of two chromatids attached at a centromere. The length of chromosomes and position of the centromere (metacentric, acrocentric) are used to classify chromosomes. An ordered array of chromosome photographic images is a karyotype in which 23 pairs will be found in the normal preparation. Abnormal numbers, extra chromosomes (polyploidy) and missing or broken chromosomes (aneuploidy) can be readily established. ($\times$4,200)

Figure 2.   Electron micrograph of cell in telophase. The chromosomes (Ch) appear as two large masses of electron-dense granular material moving toward pairs of centrioles (Ce) positioned at each cell pole. The plasma membrane (PM) is invaginated at the equatorial plate, indicative of initiation of cleavage of the dividing cell into daughter cells. Some mitochondria are seen in the equatorial midbody region and about the centrioles. ($\times$10,300)

Figure 3.   Electron micrograph of chromosome at one cell pole. Four stages are usually named in describing the mitotic activity of a cell: prophase, metaphase, anaphase, and telophase which is illustrated here. Most of the cell life is spent in interphase. This is subdivided into a G1 phase which follows completion of mitosis in which no DNA synthesis occurs, an S phase in which DNA synthesis occurs until the DNA is exactly doubled, and a G2 phase preceding mitosis in which no more DNA synthesis occurs. At prophase, chromosomes are discrete and consist of two closely approximated chromatids. The chromosomes are attached at a constriction, the centromere. The nucleolus and nuclear membrane disappear. At metaphase, the mitotic apparatus is formed in which centriole pairs (Ce) are related by their satellites (S) to microtubules (SF) about 20 to 27 mμ in diameter attached to the chromosome at the centromere. Other microtubules course from one pole to the other without attaching to chromosomes. These are the central continuous tubules. The centriole pairs occupy each pole of the cell and the chromosomes occupy the equatorial plate. Cytoplasmic elements including mitochondria, ribosomes (Ri) and various vesicles (Ve) are distributed around the chromosomes and cell poles. Centromeres have divided during metaphase, and in anaphase each chromatid, now a single chromosome, is moved by the microtubules toward the cell poles. At telophase, the chromosomes approach the cell poles and the nucleolus and nuclear envelope reappear, the chromosomes uncoil and cytokinesis occurs. ($\times$38,500)

PLATE 13

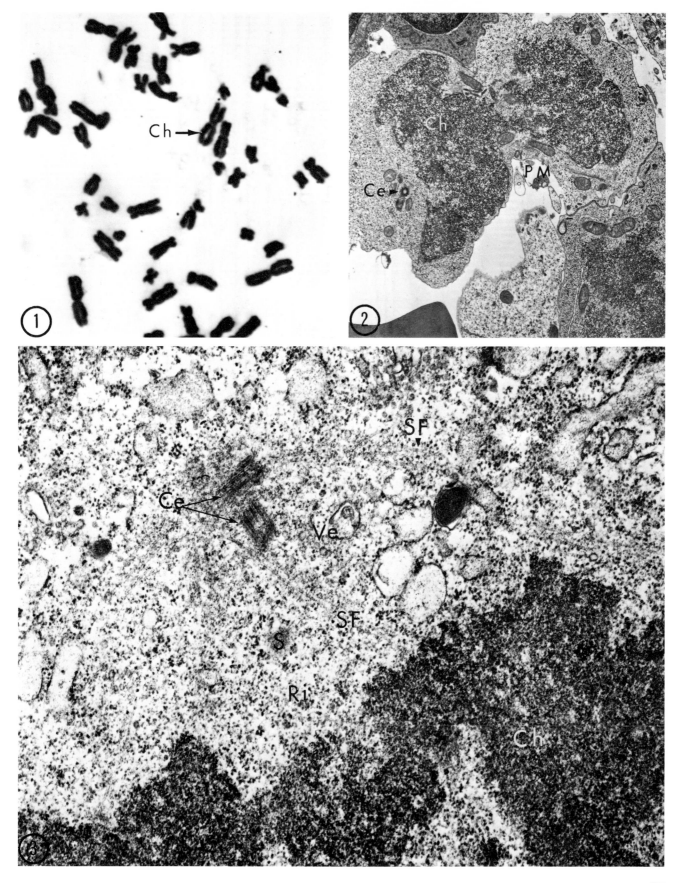

Epithelium

Plate 14 — SIMPLE SQUAMOUS
EPITHELIUM

Figure 1. Photomicrograph of kidney cortex. The glomerulus of the kidney consists of an outer parietal (Pa) layer of epithelial cells separated from a visceral layer of epithelial cells by a capsular space (CS) which receives the plasma filtrate. The visceral epithelial cells surround the capillaries (V) of the glomerular tuft. All three of these epithelial layers are simple squamous. The term *endothelium* is used for the lining cells of the vascular system while the term *epithelium* is used for the others. The term *mesothelium* is applied to squamous cells covering the visceral organs. These simple squamous cells have a flat profile which bulges at the nucleus (N). ($\times$570)

Figure 2. Photomicrograph of epon-embedded kidney. Simple squamous endothelium is seen in profile lining a vessel (V). A thin loop (TL) of a nephron is lined with simple squamous epithelium. The cytoplasm is thin and appears as a fine line which bulges at the nucleus. Simple cuboidal epithelium (SC) comprises the walls of adjacent tubules. ($\times$190)

Figure 3. Electron micrograph of simple squamous endothelial cells of a vessel wall. The plasma membranes are separated by sparse amounts of cytoplasm. Occasionally the membranes have thin windows called fenestrae, which are spherical when viewed from the surface (see Plate 131). Pinocytotic vesicles (PV) may be found at the plasma membrane at either side of the cell. A junction (CJ) between two endothelial cells shows a desmosomal-type complex. Extensions of the two cells project for a short distance into the lumen at the junction site. Some junctions may show overlapping of adjacent cells. Mitochondria and rough-surfaced endoplasmic reticulum are sparse. A thin basal lamina (BL) separates these cells from the surrounding connective tissue (CT). ($\times$10,700)

Insert. Photomicrograph of surface view of simple squamous epithelium. In this view, the cells appear platelike in shape with a central nucleus. ($\times$240)

30

PLATE 14

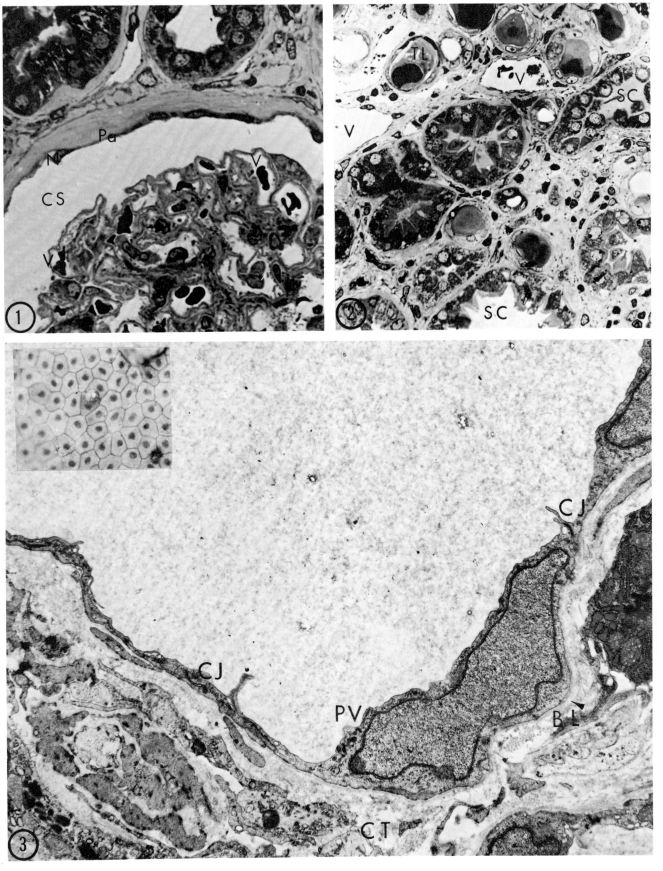

Plate 15 — SIMPLE CUBOIDAL EPITHELIUM

Figure 1. Photomicrograph of kidney tubules. The lumina (L) of these tubules seen in cross section are bounded by a single layer of cells the outer basal surfaces of which rest upon a basal lamina (BL). The nuclei of these cells are positioned centrally. In some instances, the plasma membrane can be seen between adjacent cells; it is often hard to see, however, and the membrane position is estimated. The cell width and length are similar, i.e. cuboidal. In instances where the length slightly exceeds the width, the term *low columnar* is applied. Smaller tubules in the field are lined with simple squamous epithelium (SS). Capillaries (C) are lined with simple squamous endothelium. (×375)

Figure 2. Photomicrograph of thyroid follicles. In this view, the nuclei of the cuboidal cells comprising the walls of the follicles (F) are oval. The membranes between adjacent cells are obscure but can be estimated by noting the nuclear position of adjacent cells. The cytoplasm of some of these cells is thin, presumably due to filling of the follicle with colloid. (×375)

Figure 3. Electron micrograph of cuboidal cells of thyroid follicle. The nuclei (N) of these cells are round and show a finely condensed chromatin. The apical portions of the cells show small microvilli (Mv) projecting into the colloid (Col) within the follicle. The apical end of the cell may be slightly narrower than the basal part, which is folded and rests upon a basal lamina (BL). Junctional complexes (TJ) anchor adjacent cells at their apices. Mitochondria (M), vesicles of varying density, and a Golgi complex (G) are seen in the apical cytoplasm. Some mitochondria and vesicles (V) occupy the basal cytoplasm. Free ribosomes (Ri) and polyribosomes are randomly distributed. The rough-surfaced endoplasmic reticulum is dilated into large cisternae, (C). (×7,000)

PLATE 15

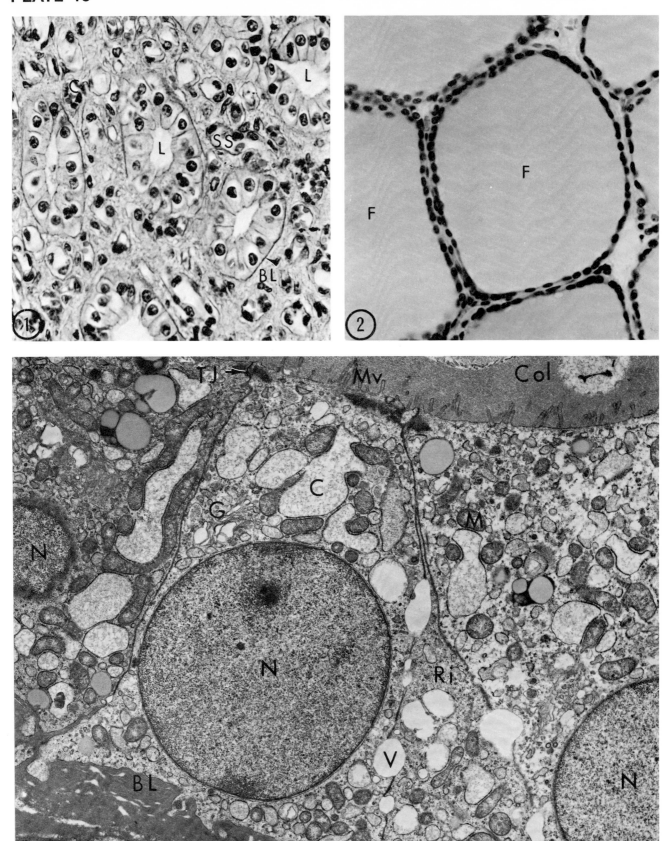

Plate 16 — SIMPLE COLUMNAR EPITHELIUM

Figure 1. Photomicrograph of simple columnar epithelium of small intestine. This epithelium consists of a single row of elongated cells resting upon a basal lamina (BL). The cell portion adjacent to the lamina is the basal portion while the portion adjacent to the lumen is referred to as the apical portion. Each cell has an elongated nucleus (N) situated in the basal part. These cells show a polarity such that secretory products in the form of mucin droplets are localized in the apical portion. A fine striated border (SB) consisting of microvilli characterizes the plasma membrane at the apex. ($\times$375)

Figure 2. Photomicrograph of epon-embedded pyloric gland. These cells also show a basal nuclear polarity. The cells are long and narrow with a striated border (SB). The epithelium is separated from the subjacent connective tissue by a basal lamina (BL). ($\times$375)

Figure 3. Electron micrograph of simple columnar epithelial cells from mucous neck cell region of fundic stomach. The cells rest upon a basal lamina (BL). The nuclei (N) occupy the basal portion and contain prominent nucleoli (Nu). The cytoplasm contains mitochondria (M), rough endoplasmic reticulum (ER) and a Golgi complex (G) on the apical side of the nucleus. Mucin droplets (Mu) are clustered at the apex and appear as spherules of moderate density sometimes containing globules of greater density. The cell surface shows some small microvilli (Mv). Other columnar cells may show neither mucin nor secretory granules and may serve principally as lining or absorptive cells. ($\times$7,400)

PLATE 16

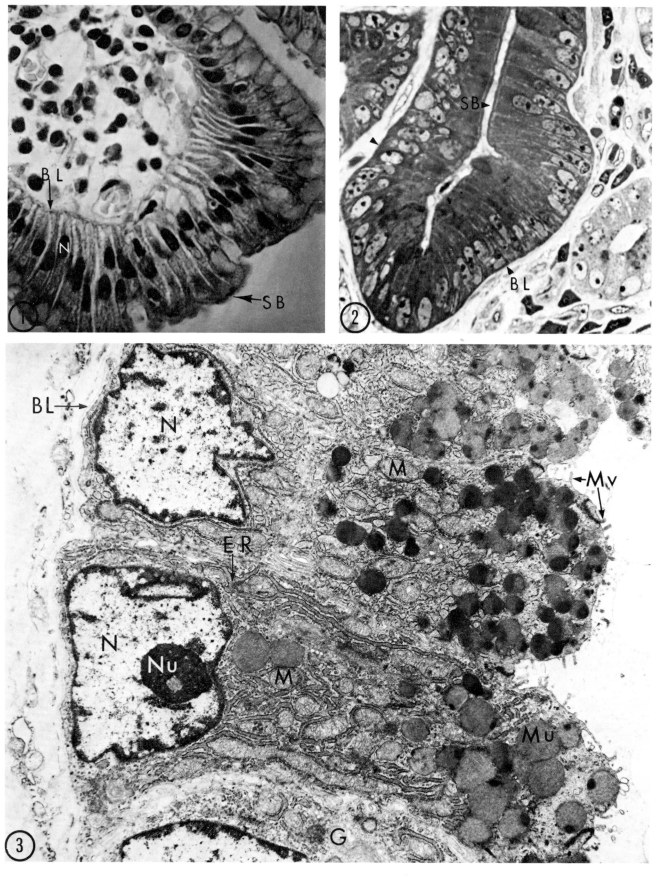

Plate 17 — GOBLET CELL AND JUNCTIONAL COMPLEXES

Figure 1. Electron micrograph of microvilli of intestinal lining cell. The surface of the microvilli is coated with a mucinous glycocalyx (Gx). Each microvillus (Mv) is limited by the plasma membrane and contains electron-dense filaments (arrow) continuous with the filaments of the terminal web (TW) lying at the base of the microvilli. These filaments apparently give some support to the microvilli. Tubules have also been described in the core of microvilli, and it is suggested that they serve to transport absorbed materials to the cell interior. (×51,000)

Figure 2. Electron micrograph of goblet cell (GC) and adjacent lining columnar cells. The lumen surface of the goblet cell is devoid of microvilli and protrudes into the lumen. This protrusion and the distended shape of the middle of the cell are due to the retention of mucus-containing spherules. Secretion is effected by a rupture of the plasma membrane at the lumen, resulting in the sudden collapse of the cell and extrusion of its contents into the lumen. The microvilli (Mv) of the adjacent cells show a herringbone pattern due to the tangential direction of section. (×6,400)

Figure 3. Electron micrograph of the junctional complex of two lining columnar cells. The plasma membrane covering the microvilli (Mv) continues between the two adjacent cells. The membranes of the two cells are closely apposed along the entire cell length, but certain special modifications occur. Very close to the lumen the outer dark layer of each individual plasma membrane (which ordinarily appears in electron micrographs as two dark lines separated by a lipid-rich space) fuses with the outer membrane of the adjacent cell membrane, effectively blocking any movement of substances between cells. This line of fusion occurs only a short distance along the membranes and is called a zonula occludens (ZO). This selective membrane fusion circles each cell and may be likened to a belt. The membranes are slightly separated below this fusion site, sometimes referred to as a "tight junction." A second attachment is then formed also completely encircling each cell. This second attachment point is the macula occludens (MO) and differs from the zonula occludens in that the membranes are not actually fused. Each plasma membrane still retains a definitive three-layer appearance. An electron-dense material can be seen between the adjacent plasma membranes and, additionally, an electron-dense material is observed on the cytoplasmic side of this adhesion point. Tonofibrils (Tf) project into the cytoplasm from these points. A third adhesion structure may be seen at any lower point on the adjacent membranes. This structure is called the macula adherens (MA) and occurs elsewhere as desmosomes. These structures show the same layers as the macula but occur only in localized areas. They do not completely encircle the cell, and thus any plane of section will not necessarily include desmosomes. (×64,000)

PLATE 17

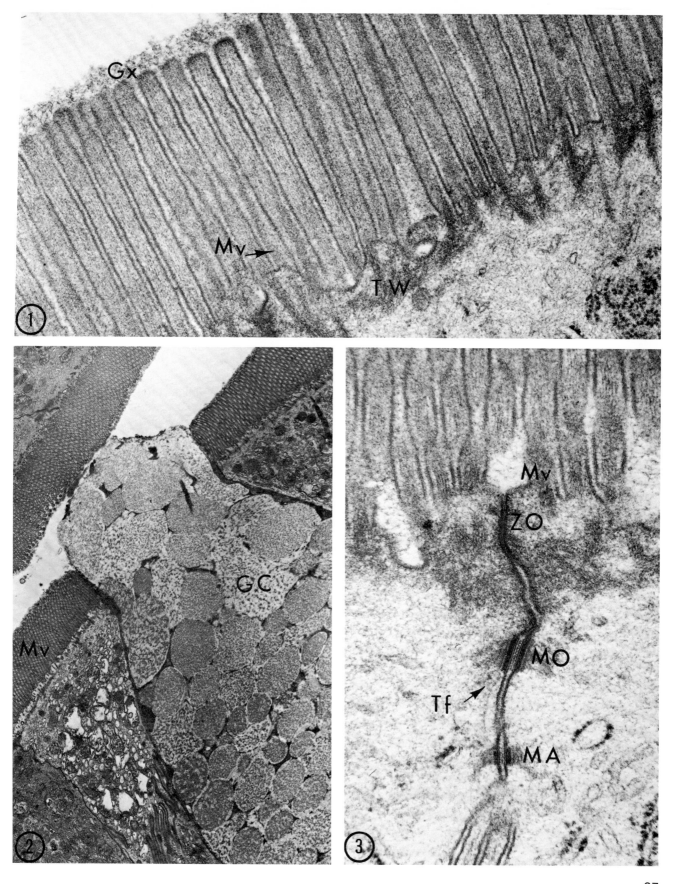

Plate 18 — PSEUDOSTRATIFIED COLUMNAR EPITHELIUM

Figure 1.   Pseudostratified columnar epithelium consists of several cell types. At least two levels of nuclei are present. Large ovoid nuclei are situated close to the lumen in cells with cytoplasm extending to the lumen, and smaller nuclei are located in the basal region of adjacent cells which do not readily reach the lumen. These cells rest upon a prominent basal lamina (BL). The staggered levels of nuclei give the illusion of a stratified epithelium, particularly in tangential sections. (×320)

Figure 2.   Ciliated pseudostratified columnar epithelium. In this section from the covering of the pharyngeal tonsil, the two types of nuclei are readily distinguished. Large nuclei are pale staining and small nuclei are basophilic. Fine filamentous structures, the cilia, are present on the lumen cell surface. The basal lamina is not prominent in this organ. The subjacent tissue consists of randomly dispersed developing lymphoid cells. (×400)

Figure 3.   Electron micrograph of apical portion of three cells of ciliated pseudostratified columnar epithelium. In this view, cilia are seen to contain internal filaments (F) encased in an outfolding of the plasma membrane (PM). The filaments arise from a basal body (BB) having the structure of a centriole. A cross-striated filamentous foot process extends from the basal body into the cytoplasm. This is shown associated with the cilia depicted in Plate 122. Mitochondria (M) are prominent in these cells. Some free ribosomes and smooth endoplasmic reticulum are also present. The plasmalemma of adjacent cells fuse at their apical points of contact to form "tight junctions" (T). (×21,500)

PLATE 18

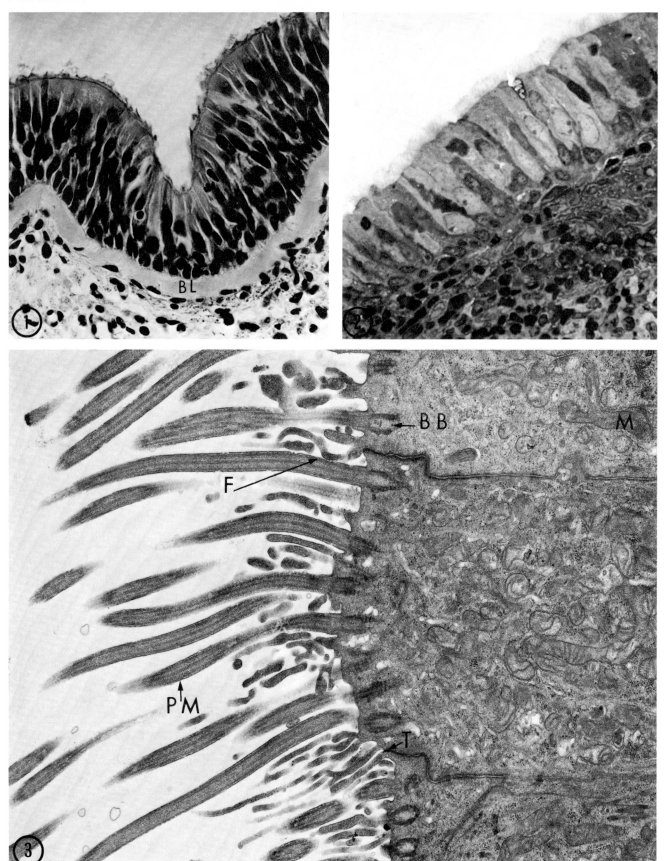

Plate 19 — STRATIFIED SQUAMOUS EPITHELIUM

Figure 1. Photomicrograph of skin. Stratified squamous epithelium (SS) covers the body and lines all structures opening to the outside: the mouth, nasal vestibule, anus, external auditory canal, vagina, etc. This epithelium varies in thickness, depending primarily upon the effects of drying, pressure, or friction. Areas subject to trauma have an outer surface of keratin (K). This epithelium consists of several cell layers, continuously replaced by generations of new cells at the basal region and desquamation of old cells and keratin at the free surface. The tissue below the epithelium is dense fibrous irregular connective tissue (CT) in which the intercellular material is more abundant than the cells. ($\times$100)

Figure 2. Photomicrograph of epon-embedded stratified squamous epithelium. The epithelial cells rest upon a basal lamina (BL). The cells are cuboidal at the lamina and change to spinous cells (SC) in the next layer. The cells closest to the free surface are squamous shaped (SS). The shape of the surface cells of stratified epithelia is used to classify the epithelium. A layer of keratin (K), the proteinaceous product of these cells, covers the free surface. Cells in the connective tissue (CT) are fibroblasts. ($\times$375)

Figure 3. Electron micrograph of stratum corneum of skin. Stratified squamous epithelium is too thick to permit a view of the entire width at this magnification. Other views of the characteristic strata of squamous epithelium may be found in Plates 146 and 149. The cells included here, from the stratum corneum, show the typical flattened platelike shape of squamous cells seen in profile. The nucleus (N) has clumped chromatin and a nucleolus (Nu). As the cells are pushed closer to the surface as new cells are generated, their nuclei become smaller and denser (pyknotic) and ultimately are destroyed by karyolysis. The cytoplasm contains few organelles but is filled with tonofibrils (Tf). The plasma membranes of contiguous cells are close, and have small processes united at desmosomes (D). ($\times$6,900)

PLATE 19

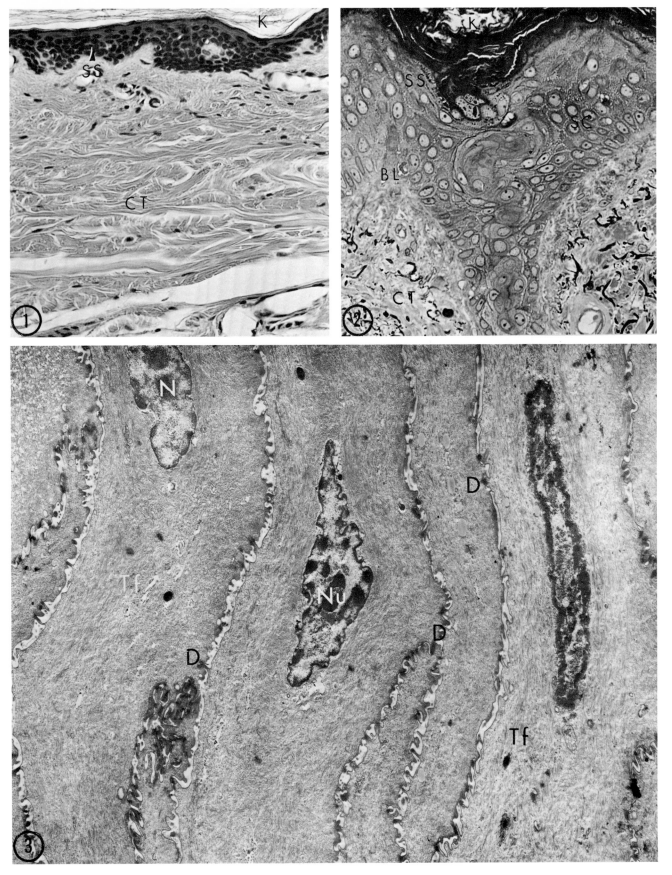

Plate 20 — TRANSITIONAL EPITHELIUM

Figure 1. Photomicrograph of transitional epithelium of urinary bladder. This epithelium is presumed to vary in thickness from a minimum of four layers of cells when the bladder is distended to ten layers when the bladder is empty. The outermost cells of the epithelium (E) are usually pear shaped or rounded, but cuboidal cells have been found mixed with round ones particularly in the transitional epithelium of the ureter. This is a stratified epithelium but the word *stratified* is ordinarily omitted from the classification, possibly because there is no simple counterpart. The epithelium rests upon a basal lamina (BL) which may be intermittently fenestrated. (×500)

Figure 2. Electron micrograph of transitional epithelium. The transitional epithelial cells reaching the lumen (L) of the urinary system are pear shaped and may be binucleated (N). The nucleus contains a prominent nucleolus (Nu). The nuclear envelope has numerous fenestrae. Large amounts of glycogen (Gl) are dispersed in the cytoplasm among free ribosomes (Ri). Mitochondria (M) are small and tubular. Occasional membranes of both rough- and smooth-surfaced endoplasmic reticulum are found. Some surface cells are smaller and darker, and contain pyknotic nuclei. Degenerative changes in the cytoplasm may be observed, as seen in the cell marked DC, suggesting that continuous death and replacement of lining cells occur. A limited number of small microvilli project into the lumen. Tight junctions (TJ) and desmosomes join the cells, even though considerable distortion and "slipping" of cells apparently occur during bladder distension. The apparent thinness of this epithelium seen with the light microscope in some instances may be illusory. (×5,800)

Figure 3. Electron micrograph of transitional epithelium. The epithelial cells are separated from the underlying connective tissue collagen (Co) by a thin interrupted basal lamina (BL). The epithelial cells vary in density and content. The nuclei (N) have finely condensed chromatin and contain a large nucleolus. The nuclei are round but may have a large cleft. The cytoplasm of basal cells contains an abundance of ribosomes (Ri). The mitochondria (M) are oval or tubular and contain many more cristae than the mitochondria of the superficial cell. The cytoplasm of adjacent cells is adapted to fit so that little intercellular space is present. Some cells show a more folded basal plasma membrane (P), have smaller and more granular nuclei, and contain many lysosomes (L). These basal cells contain fewer free ribosomes but have more rough-surfaced endoplasmic reticulum (ER). A small Golgi complex (G) is present. (×9,500)

42

PLATE 20

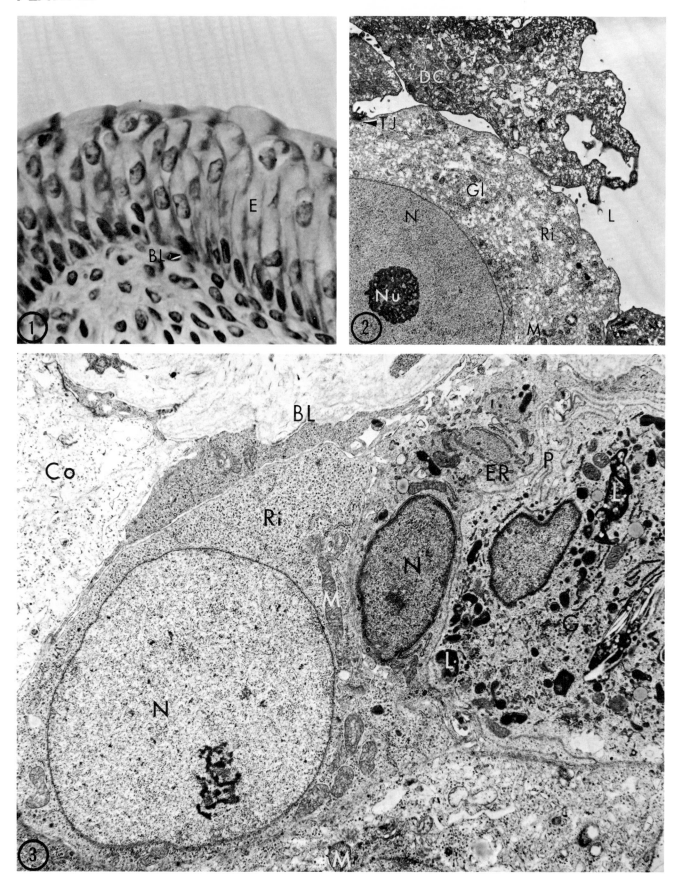

Connective and
Supporting Tissue

PLATE 27

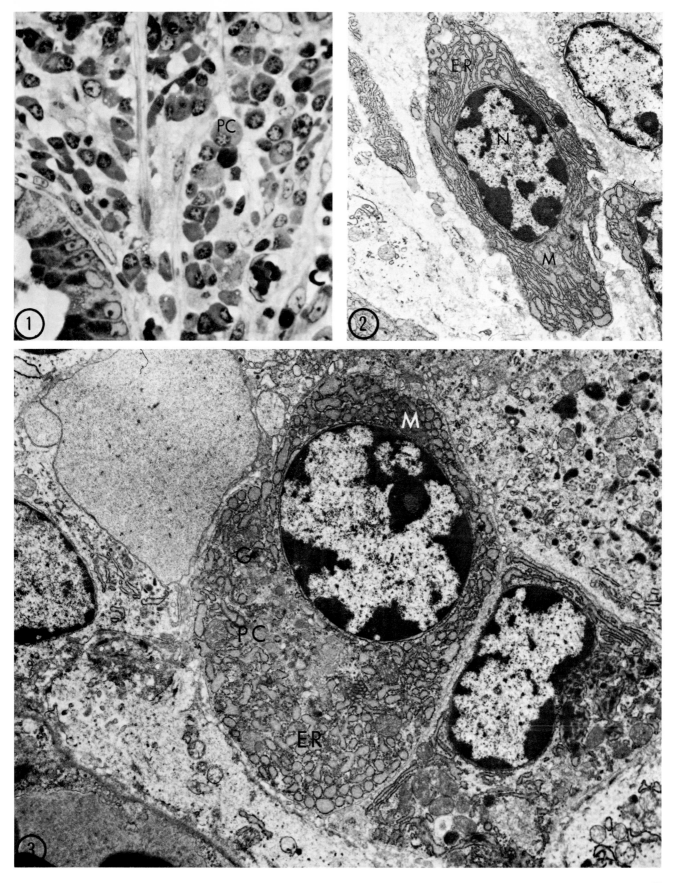

Plate 28 — MELANOCYTE

Figure 1.   Photomicrograph of epidermis. The cytoplasm of some of the basal cells of the epithelium (BC) contains granules. These granules are produced by melanocytes located at the base of the epithelial cells or inserted between them. Melanocytes have long slender processes between epithelial cells, providing a ready means of transfer of granules from melanocyte to epithelial cell. Prior to synthesizing melanin, melanocytes often appear as clear cells (Mc) at the basal lamina. A positive identification can be made with the dopa reaction demonstrating the presence of tyrosinase, an enzyme essential for melanin production. ($\times$400)

Figure 2.   Photomicrograph of epon-embedded section of iris. The epithelial cells (EC) on the posterior surface of the iris contain large melanin granules which they produce. Scattered in the connective tissue stroma (St) of the iris are capillaries (C), smooth muscle fibers (SM), fibroblasts (F), and pigment-containing melanocytes (Me). These cells have an irregular shape, extend long processes, and contain melanin granules smaller than those seen in the epithelial cells. ($\times$375)

Figure 3.   Electron micrograph of melanocyte in skin. The stratified squamous epithelium of the skin (SS) rests upon an intact basal lamina (BL). Collagen (Co) and elastic fibers (EF) are randomly oriented below the basal lamina. A melanocyte is located about 15 μ from the basal lamina and extends several processes in that direction. It has a finely granular nucleus (N) with an irregular shape. Melanosomes in the form of membrane-bound clusters of melanin crystals and lamellae are located in the epithelial side of the cytoplasm and are associated with a large Golgi apparatus (G). ($\times$8,800)

60

PLATE 28

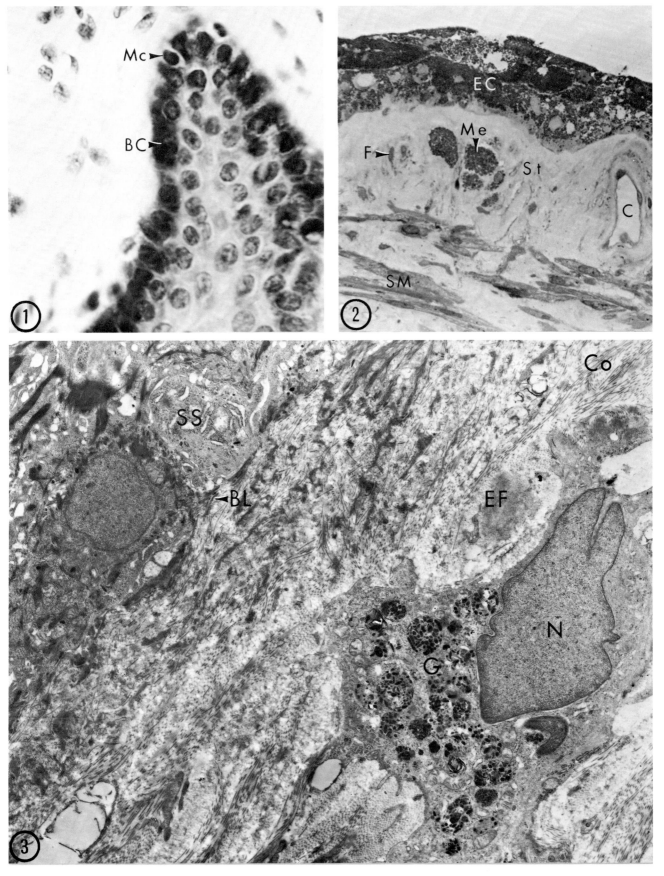

Plate 29 — GROWTH PLATE

Figure 1. Photomicrograph of cartilaginous epiphysis. The cartilage growth plate and the articular cartilage of bone are hyaline cartilage, characterized by an apparent afibrillar glassy matrix surrounding the chondrocytes (C). In the growth plate, a progression of changes occurs. In a growth plate separated on one side by marrow of the epiphysis and on the other by marrow of the metaphysis, the cells are arranged in columns parallel to the bone axis. The first cells at the epiphysis are called resting cells. Deep to this cell layer are flattened chondroblasts dividing mitotically. Several cells may occupy one lacuna. This is the zone of proliferation (P). Deep to this zone the cells are larger and are separated by newly synthesized matrix, the zone of matrix synthesis (MS). Chondrocytes in columns then become hypertrophic (H) and the matrix mineralizes along these cells in the zone of provisional calcification (PC). Cartilage cell death follows this event and the empty lacunae serve as bone formation sites. ($\times 375$)

Figure 2. Electron micrograph of longitudinal section of chondrocyte in zone of proliferation. The cells in this zone are flattened, contain elongated nuclei (N) and have several thin cytoplasmic extensions. Mitotic forms are best seen in transverse sections through this zone. The cells contain glycogen inclusions (Gl) and rough-surfaced endoplasmic reticulum (ER). They occupy a lacuna bounded by a finely fibrillar matrix consisting of collagen filaments and amorphous ground substance. Both matrix components are synthesized by these cells. ($\times 5,100$)

Figure 3. Electron micrograph of chondrocyte from zone of matrix synthesis. The cell is larger and has a central nucleus (N). A large Golgi complex (G) is located adjacent to the nucleus. Several secretion vesicles (V) are associated with the Golgi complex and may also be seen at the plasma membrane. These presumably contain tropocollagen molecules and mucopolysaccharide. Mitochondria (M), glycogen (Gl), and rough-surfaced endoplasmic reticulum (ER) are distributed randomly in the cytoplasm. The plasma membrane is extended around narrow processes which may reach through the matrix to processes of adjacent cells. ($\times 22,000$)

PLATE 29

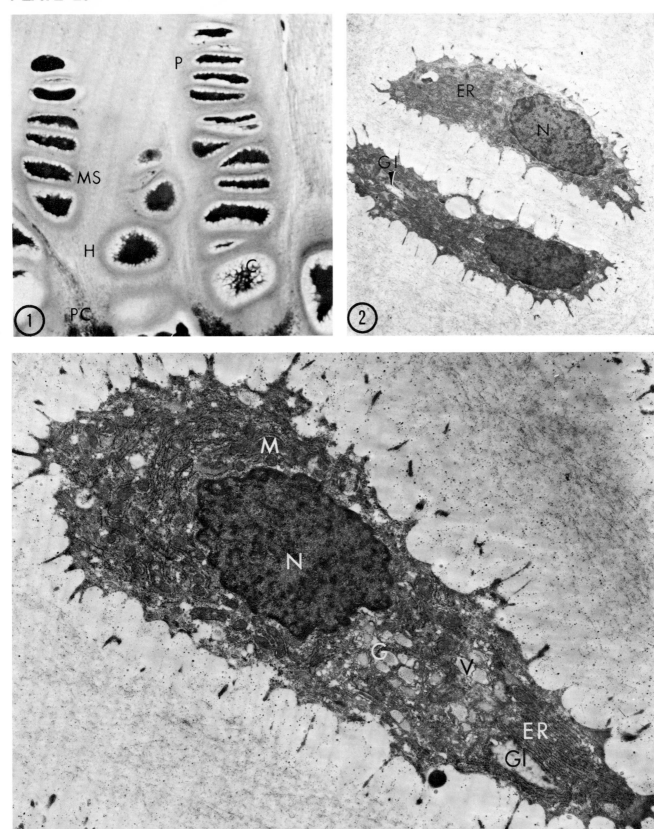

Plate 30 — GROWTH PLATE

Figure 1.   Photomicrograph of epon-embedded cartilaginous epiphysis. The resting zone (RZ), zone of proliferation (ZP), zone of matrix synthesis (MS), hypertrophy (H), and provisional calcification (PC) are indicated. It can be noted that the longitudinal column walls are mineralized while the transverse septa become thin. Erythrocytes (E) and osteoblasts are seen on the metaphyseal surface. ($\times 375$)

Figure 2.   Electron micrograph of matrix from zone of provisional calcification. In this zone, the collagen fibrils are compressed and are larger than those in the younger zones. Some fibers are large enough to demonstrate axial periodicity. The mineral phase first appears as round clusters of hydroxy apatite crystals (A) which later coalesce to form a solid mineral trabeculum. ($\times 34,000$)

Figure 3.   Electron micrograph of chondrocyte from zone of cell hypertrophy. A large Golgi complex (G) occupies a juxtanuclear (N) position. Mitochondria (M) and rough-surfaced endoplasmic reticulum (ER) are widely scattered. Numerous vesicles and some microbodies (L) are present. A cilium (C) extends into the matrix. The cell is large. The plasma membrane has several processes, giving the cell surface a scalloped appearance. The organelles are reduced in number, the nucleus becomes pyknotic, and the plasma membrane is attenuated in the lower zones. ($\times 11,800$)

PLATE 30

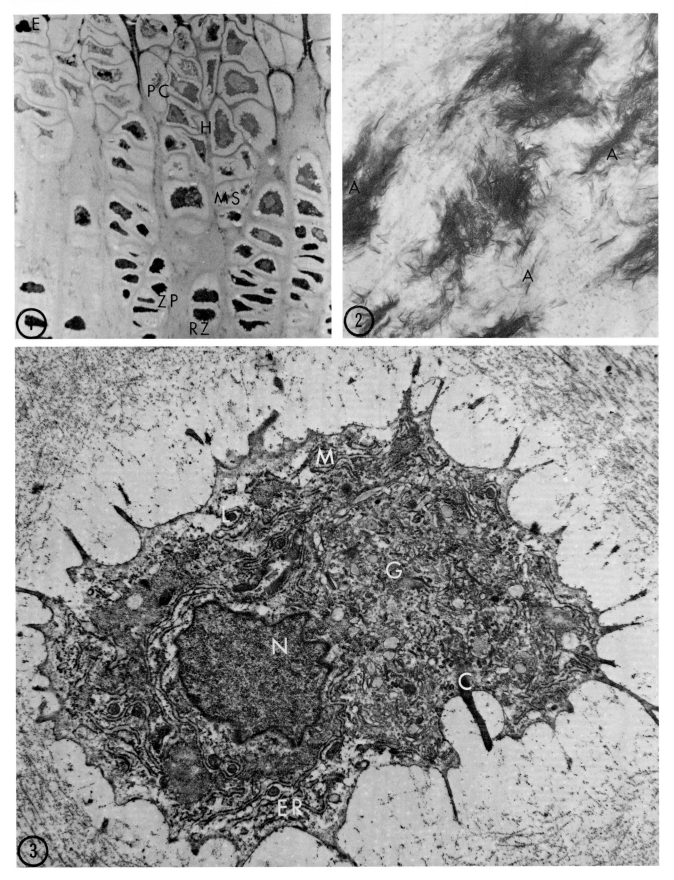

Plate 31 — OSTEOBLAST

Figure 1. Photomicrograph of medullary space in bone. The endosteal surface (E) is lined by a single continuous row of osteoblasts (Ob). Osteocytes (Oc) in lacunar spaces communicate with the osteoblasts by processes extended into the canaliculi (arrows). Fluid surrounding the osteoblasts circulates around the canalicular processes and reaches the lacunar spaces. ($\times$375)

Figure 2. Photomicrograph of demineralized epon-embedded bone. A medullary space (M) is lined by osteoblasts (Ob) at the bone (B) surface. Osteocytes (Oc) occupy the lacunae (L). ($\times$375)

Figure 3. Electron micrograph of osteoblasts. The osteoblasts covering bone may be flattened and contain few organelles or they may be cuboidal in shape and contain several organelles. This variation in morphology may indicate periods of new synthesis of matrix components and periods of quiescence. Cells in the latter stage have been called "lining cells" by some investigators. The mineralized bone (B) is electron dense. A collagenous matrix of osteoid (Os) separates the mineralized bone from the osteoblast. The distal side of the osteoblast is adjacent to marrow cells and blood vessels and becomes surrounded by osteoid only when extensive growth of new bone occurs, committing the cell to become an entrapped osteocyte. These cells contain mitochondria (M), rough-surfaced endoplasmic reticulum (ER), and small vesicles. A Golgi apparatus is usually present but is not included in this plane of section. Numerous small cell processes (P) extend into the osteoid. Pinocytotic vesicles (PV) may be found on both sides of the cell. Membranes of adjacent cells may be as close as 10 mμ but desmosomes or tight junctions are not common features. Cells are often widely separated. Continuity of tissue fluid on the capillary side with fluid on the bone side and in the lacunar spaces has been established with horseradish peroxidase, a protein which migrates rapidly between these cells. ($\times$8,700)

PLATE 31

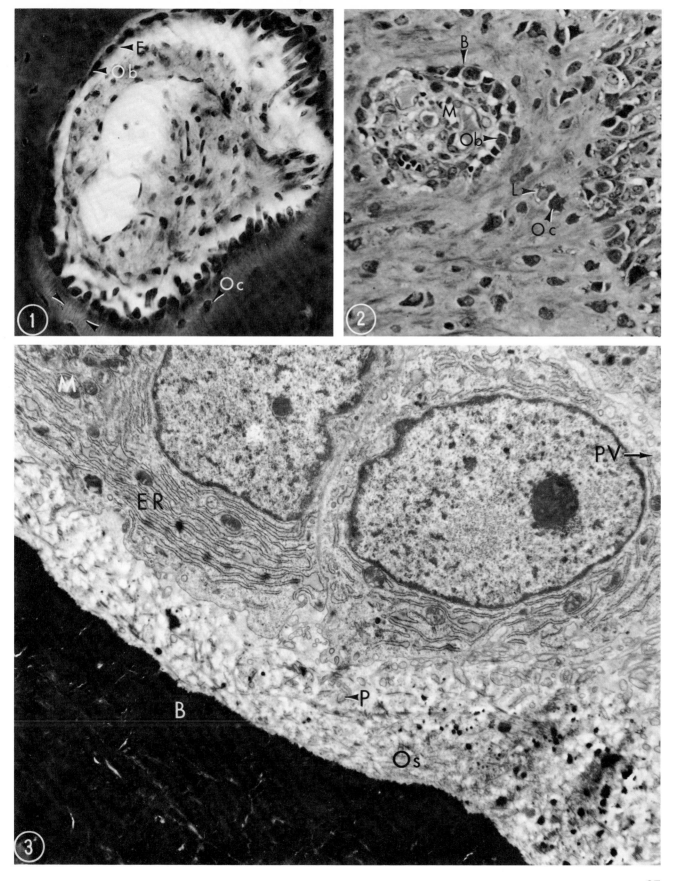

Plate 32 – OSTEOCYTE

Figure 1. Photomicrograph of compact bone. Compact bone is composed of lamellae of mineralized bone matrix separated by a cement line. These lamellae are arranged in sheets which follow the contour of the inner (endosteal) (E) and outer (periosteal) (P) surfaces. Special tubular systems occupy the middle zones. Blood vessels coursing longitudinally through the bone are surrounded by several lamellae resembling a series of pipes slipped one inside the other. This arrangement is a haversian system (HS). Irregular lamellae sandwiched between haversian lamellae are called interstitial lamellae. Integral parts of these lamellae are the osteocytes (O) which occupy lacunar spaces in the matrix. The lacunae of all lamellae are connected by canaliculi through which processes of osteocytes are extended. ($\times$60)

Figure 2. Electron micrograph of young osteocyte. Bone forms by apposition of new matrix (osteoid) upon surfaces of cartilage or bone by the synthetic activity of the osteoblasts. At regular intervals some osteoblasts become separated from the subjacent myeloid tissues by osteoid, trapping the osteoblast in a lacuna. In this figure, mineralized bone is seen in the upper left. The axial periodicity of the matrix collagen can be observed, even in the mineralized part. The mineralized bone surface is irregular, due to the presence of several new mineralizing sites (MS). A collagenous osteoid surrounds the cell. The myeloid tissue side (My) also shows some isolated initiating sites of mineralization (MS). The cell shows an abundance of rough-surfaced endoplasmic reticulum (ER), a prominent Golgi complex and several mitochondria (M), some of which contain granules. The cell surface shows the beginning of formation of processes (P) which will occupy canaliculi. ($\times$7,600).

Figure 3. Electron micrograph of young osteocyte. The mineralized bone matrix has canaliculi (Ca) into which cell processes (CP) are extended. The surrounding matrix mineralization is almost complete and the cell occupies a lacunar space (L) surrounded by osteoid (O). With entrapment within bone, synthesizing of additional matrix materials is reduced. This reduction in anabolic activity is reflected in a reduction in the number of organelles. This cell still shows a large Golgi complex (G), membranes of rough-surfaced endoplasmic reticulum (ER) and mitochondria (M). A centriole pair is included, and a cilium (Ci) extends from the centriole or basal body. A single cilium is often found on bone and cartilage cells but its significance is unknown. ($\times$10,400)

PLATE 32

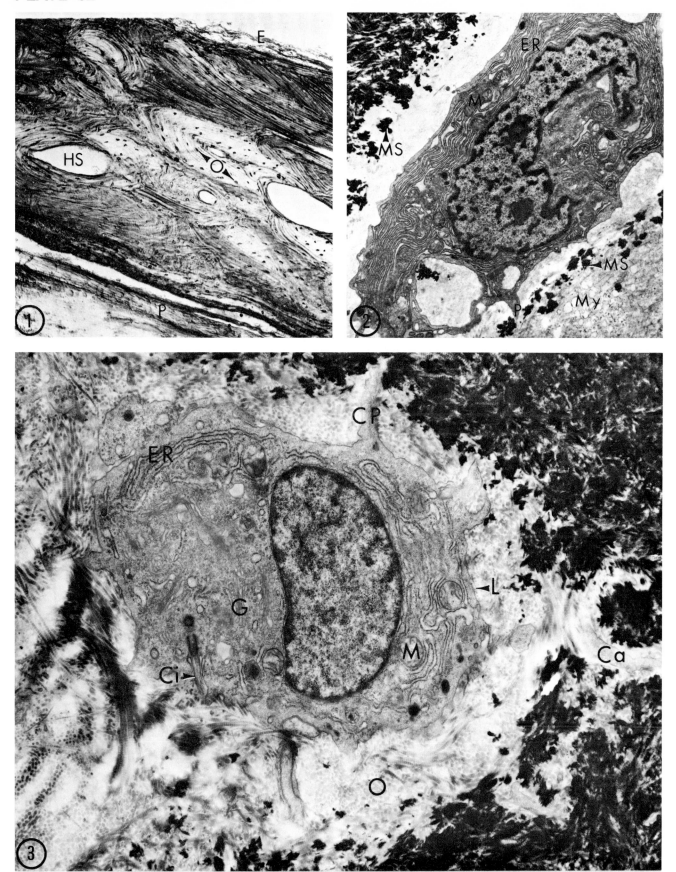

Plate 33 — OSTEOCLAST

Figure 1.   Photomicrograph of bone. Osteocytes (Oc) occupy lacunae within the bone matrix. A large resorption area is shown in the center of the field. Multinucleated osteoclasts (Ocl) occupy individual resorption concavities called Howship's lacunae. (×150)

Figure 2.   Photomicrograph of medullary bone. The endosteal surface is lined by osteoblasts (Ob) and multinucleated osteoclasts (Ocl). The osteoclast cytoplasm is basophilic. Fibroblasts, mesenchymal cells, capillaries and a fibrillar net occupy the rest of the medullary space. (×150)

Figure 3.   Electron micrograph of the bone surface portion of an osteoclast. One nucleus (N) of this cell is included in the upper corner. The mineralized bone (B) seen at the bottom of the figure shows a marked surface irregularity indicative of resorptive activity. The osteoclast plasma membrane shows extensive folding at the bone surface, producing evaginations in the form of microvilli (Mv) and invaginations which are continuous with membrane-lined cysternae (C) deep within the cell. Mitochondria (M) are the most prominent organelles. Those mitochondria closest to the resorption front contain electron-dense granules associated with the mitochondrial cristae, while those distal to this front show progressively lesser numbers of granules. These represent bound calcium and phosphate which were removed from the bone. Membranes of rough endoplasmic reticulum are sparse. Smooth-walled vesicles (V) are scattered throughout the cytoplasm. (×11,300)

PLATE 33

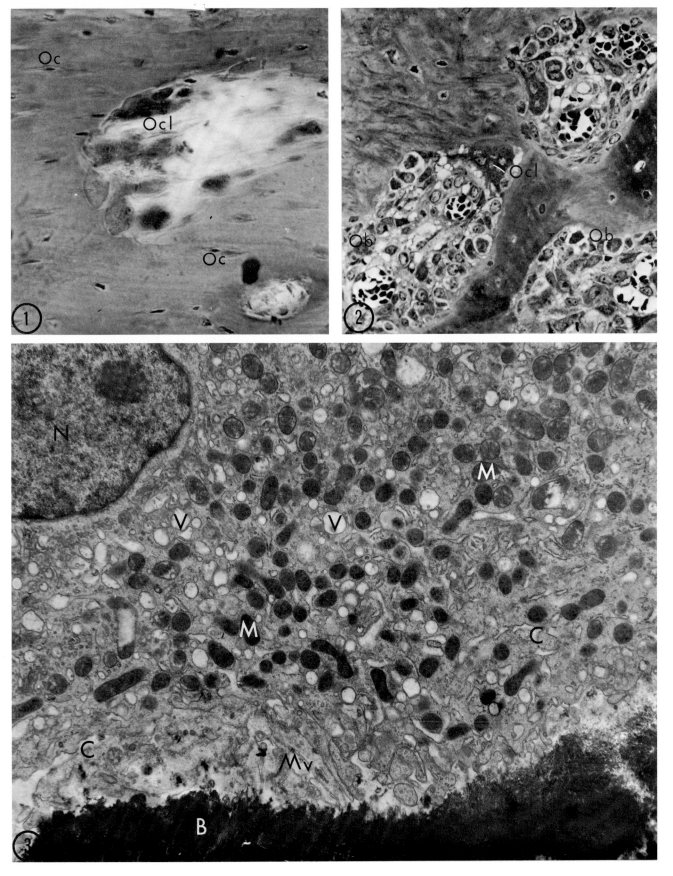

Plate 34 — ELASTIC CARTILAGE

Figure 1. Photomicrograph of elastic cartilage from larynx. Elastic cartilage differs from hyaline cartilage in the arrangement of chondrocytes (C) and in the fibrillar nature of its matrix. Numerous acidophilic elastic fibers surround each cell at the lacunar wall (LW) and course through the matrix in dense bundles. A fibrous perichondrium surrounds each cartilage plate. Lacunae are often clustered in groups such that an uneven cell distribution may be noted. (×150)

Figure 2. Electron micrograph of elastic cartilage matrix. A large elastic fiber (EF) is seen in longitudinal section. The fiber consists primarily of an amorphous electron-lucent substance, but some longitudinal filaments are buried within the amorphous elastin. Collagen fibers (Co) may form a sheath around the elastic fibers and may serve as an attachment. This sheath is not present around all elastic fibers. The surrounding matrix contains randomly oriented collagen fibers (Co). Small fibrils of elastin (El) are also present. (×16,800)

Figure 3. Electron micrograph of chondrocyte in elastic cartilage. This chondrocyte has a central nucleus (N), cytoplasm with few organelles, and a scalloped plasma membrane. Condensations of fibrillar matrix material (MM) surround the cell. The matrix is finely fibrillar and contains elastic fibers (EF) and collagen fibrils. Small electron-dense vesicles (V) are often deposited in the matrix. (×10,800)

PLATE 34

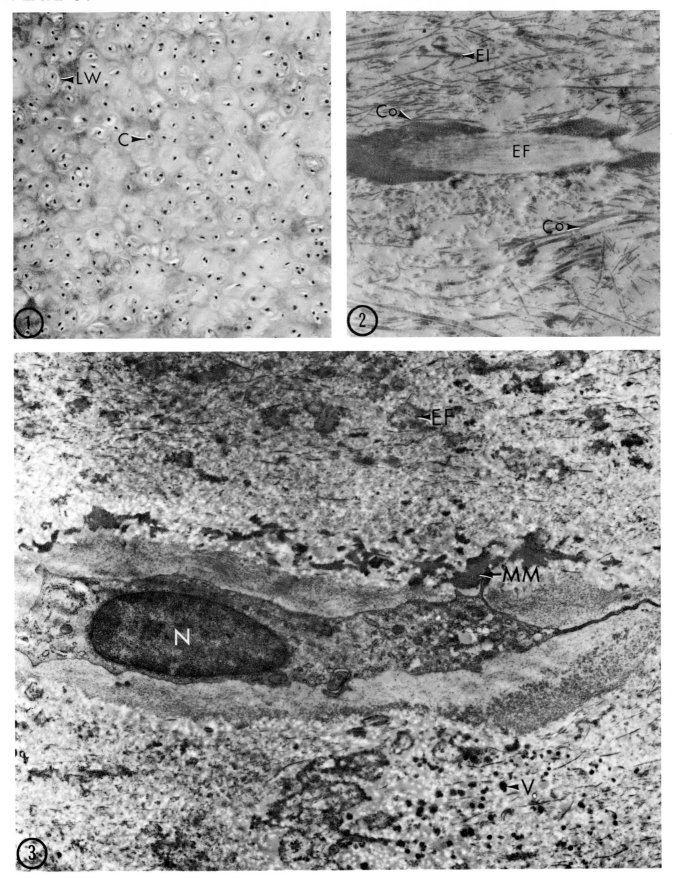

Plate 35 — FIBROCARTILAGE

Figure 1. Photomicrograph of fibrocartilage of intervertebral disc. Fibrocartilage occurs in fibrous tissues subjected to sustained pressure: the intervertebral disc, symphysis pubis and some muscle attachments. This tissue usually occurs in transition zones between regions of hyaline cartilage and dense fibrous connective tissue. In this figure, bony trabeculae (B) of the vertebral body terminate at a plate of hyaline cartilage (HC). The intervertebral disc contains large bundles of collagen fibers that course in alternate directions. Fibrocytes and some elastic fibers are also present among the fiber bundles. Intermediate between the fibrous component and the hyaline cartilage is a zone of fibrocartilage (FC). In this zone, the intercellular matrix is homogeneous and the cells occupy encapsulated lacunae (L). ($\times$120)

Figure 2. Photomicrograph of epon-embedded fibrocartilage. The chondrocytes are widely separated by matrix in fibrocartilage. Each chondrocyte is surrounded by a capsule (C) lining the walls of the lacuna. The matrix has a more fibrous appearance than hyaline cartilage. ($\times$375)

Figure 3. Electron micrograph of chondrocyte. Chondrocytes are usually elongate cells with numerous processes extending into the surrounding matrix. The nucleus is large, shows some clumping of chromatin, and is usually ovoid. The cytoplasm contains tubular-shaped mitochondria, rough-surfaced endoplasmic reticulum (ER), a large Golgi region (G). Lipid inclusions are often present. The lacuna (L) is limited by a thin fibrillar capsule. The matrix at the capsule perimeter contains an abundance of elastic fibers (EF) of varying size and density. The rest of the matrix consists of collagen fibers and ground substance. The collagen fibers are larger than those seen in hyaline cartilage and show the characteristic 64-mμ axial periodicity. ($\times$9,600)

74

PLATE 35

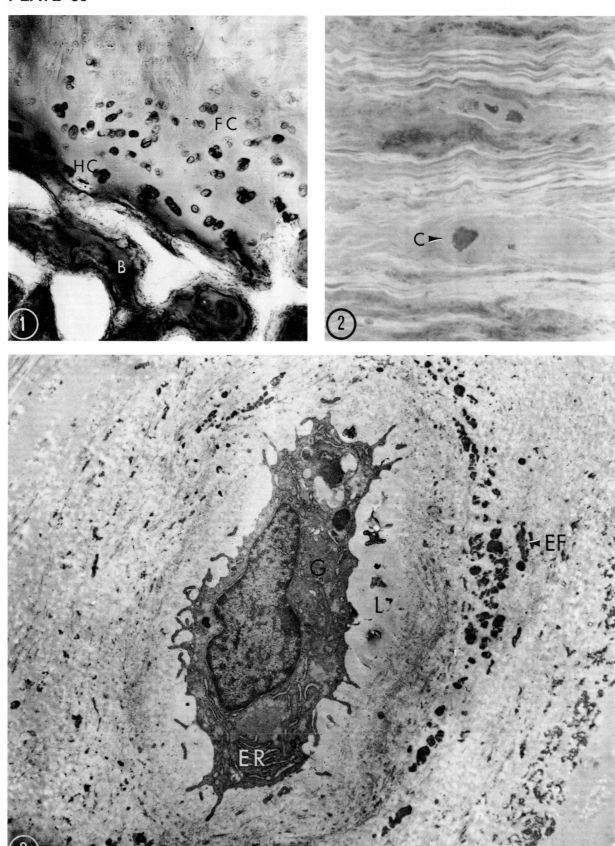

Blood and Hemopoiesis

Plate 36 — ERYTHROCYTE (RBC)

Figure 1. Photomicrograph of Wright's-stained blood smear. Mature erythrocytes (E) are anucleated biconcave discs with a diameter of about 8.5 μ in the living state. These cells retain few organelles; no centrioles, Golgi complex, or ER membranes are present. The cells are numerous, with mean values of 5.5 million per mm^3 in the male and 4.5 million per mm^3 in the female. They exhibit plasticity essential for their passage through narrow capillary channels. Erythrocytes are acidophilic and stain red pink with hemotoxylin-eosin, Wright's or Giemsa stain. ($\times$1,200)

Figure 2. Photomicrograph of erythrocytes in blood vessel. Thin sections of erythrocytes show numerous erythrocyte forms. The characteristic biconcave disc shape observed in films of intact cells is not usually seen in thin sections, as the plane of sectioning passes through the randomly positioned erythrocytes in several ways. Endothelial cells (E) line this thin-walled vein. An artery (A) with an empty lumen and kidney tubules (T) are also included in the field. ($\times$375)

Figure 3. Electron micrograph of erythrocytes. Erythrocytes (E) are osmophilic and are thus electron dense. However, formaldehyde fixative with some buffers leeches out the cytoplasm of RBCs, and the cytoplasm of cells fixed in this manner is usually a homogeneous gray. The precipitated plasma proteins give a granular pattern to the surrounding film.

The principal constituent of RBCs is hemoglobin, a protein which functions directly in the transport of oxygen but also plays a role in the transport of carbon dioxide. The hemoglobin may assume a crystalline nature in some parts of the cytoplasm. A crystal lattice of abnormal hemoglobin is characteristic of RBCs in sickle-cell anemia and is responsible for their peculiar shape in response to low oxygen tension. Ferritin granules may be seen with the hemoglobin.

Electron micrography requires thin sectioning, so the shapes seen in dried films are not usually observed. The cell membrane (PM) of RBCs has been used extensively in the study of membranes, as membrane "ghosts" of these cells are readily obtained by hemolysis of the cells in hypotonic fluids. The erythrocytes seen here appear to be stacked; a closer stacking of erythrocytes may be seen in vessels, particularly in blood which has an elevated gamma globulin. These close stacks of cells are termed rouleau formations. Young erythrocytes (reticulocytes) may enter the circulation. These cells have some internal fibrillar material best seen with brom-cresyl-blue staining. No stroma has been found in mature erythrocytes. ($\times$15,400)

PLATE 36

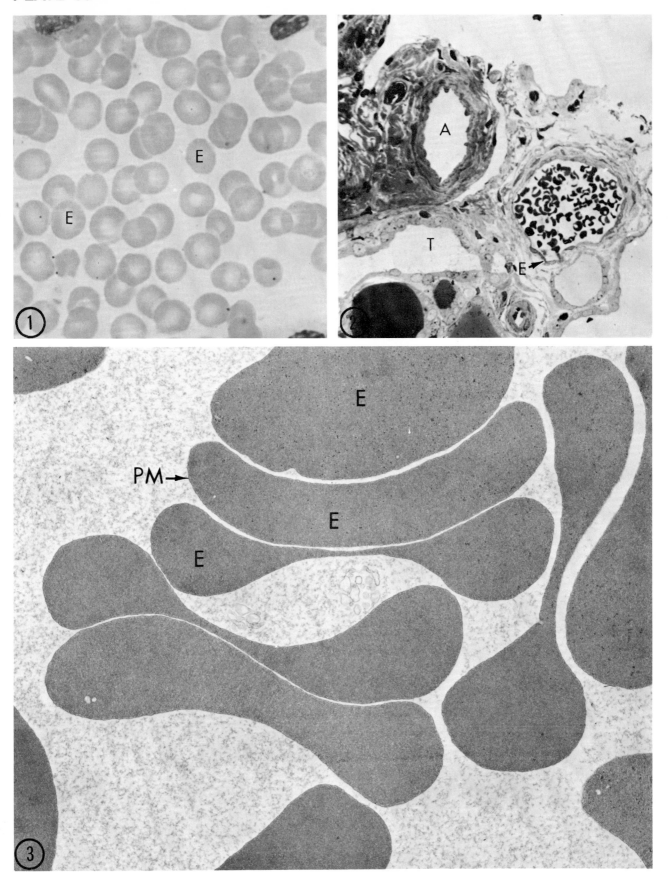

Plate 37 — ERYTHROCYTE FORMATION

Figure 1. Photomicrograph of Wright's-stained marrow smear. Erythrocytes develop in a series which progresses in the following order: reticular cells, myeloblasts (proerythroblasts), basophilic erythroblasts, polychromatophilic erythroblasts, normoblasts, reticulocytes, and erythrocytes. Most of the changes in this series are related to progressive reduction in cell size, increase in hemoglobin content, and enucleation. In this process, the nucleus undergoes size reduction and condensation, and is cast off with a slight amount of cytoplasm. Three stages are seen in this figure. The mature erythrocyte (E) is a pale-staining biconcave disc. A normocyte (N) has the size and cytoplasmic density of the erythrocytes, but contains a round pyknotic nucleus. Two larger cells, the polychromatophilic erythroblasts (PE), are so named because various hues of cytoplasm reflect different hemoglobin contents. More immature forms in the development series are seen in Figure 3. ($\times$1,160)

Figure 2. Electron micrograph of normoblast. The mature erythrocyte is an anucleate cell. In maturation, the nucleus (N) becomes condensed and is pressed to the side of the cell creating a bulge. A thin layer of cytoplasm and plasma membrane surrounds the nucleus and will be lost with the nucleus when the plasma membrane undergoes cleavage behind it. The cytoplasm of this cell contains a few mitochondria. Ferritin granules and hemoglobin give the cytoplasm its density. ($\times$14,500)

Figure 3. Electron micrograph of erythroblasts in marrow. Myeloblasts form basophilic erythroblasts (BE). These latter cells are so named because the great increase in cytoplasmic ribosomes gives the cytoplasm an intense basophilia. These cells initiate hemoglobin formation, become reduced in size and form the polychromatophilic erythroblasts (PE). The early stages have several hundred ferritin molecules scattered throughout the cytoplasm. Maturation is accompanied by reduction in amount of scattered ferritin. Excess ferritin may aggregate into vesicles and may even accumulate in mitochondria in sideroblasts. The ferritin molecule is a protein with 23% iron, octahedron shaped, with the iron at the vertices separated by about 10 mμ. Ferritin can give up its iron to hemoglobin, leaving the protein apoferritin. The iron atoms of hemoglobin are about 2.5 mμ apart; thus, hemoglobin iron and ferritin have markedly different arrangements. Ferritin enters cells of this series by a special pinocytotic process termed ropheocytosis. Succeeding cells in this series are smaller, ultimately forming normoblasts (No). The myeloblasts can also differentiate along a different cell line to form megakaryocytes or granulocytes. Parts of two cells of the neutrophil series (Ne) are also present in the field. ($\times$6,600)

PLATE 37

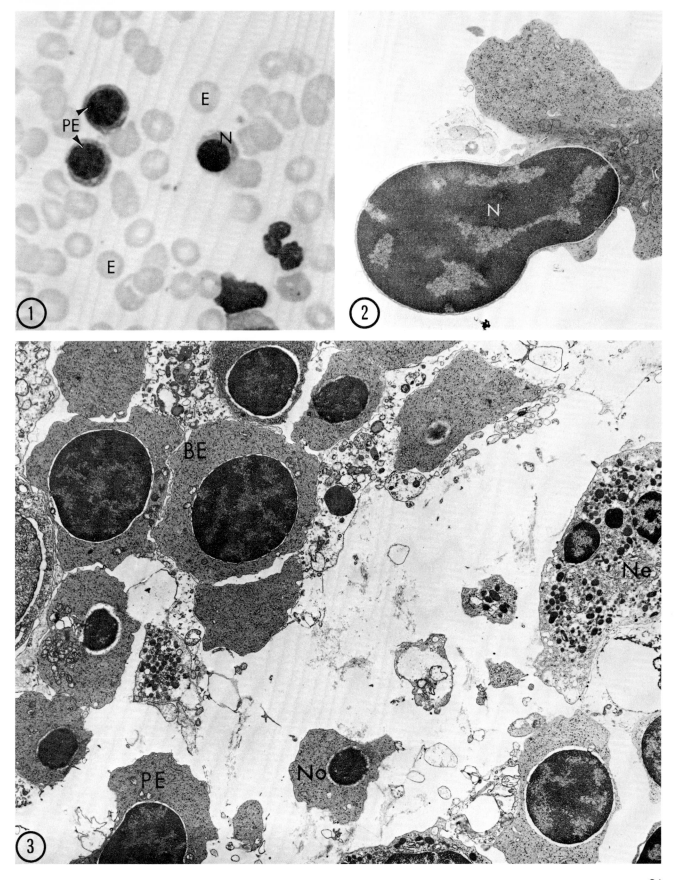

Plate 38 — NEUTROPHIL

Figure 1. Photomicrograph of Wright's-stained peripheral blood smear. Peripheral blood leukocytes are 60 to 70% neutrophils (N). The total number ranges from 3,000 to 6,500 per mm^3 of blood. Since they are the most numerous leukocytes, many may be seen in the same field, as shown here. Their diameter ranges from 10 to 12 μ. These cells are also called polymorphonucleocytes because the nucleus becomes increasingly lobed with maturation. Mature cells exhibit definite nuclear lobes connected by thin filamentous strands. Two types of granules are seen within the cytoplasm. The first to form are those staining with methylene azure and called azurophilic granules. The specific granules form later; they are small and stain faintly blue to pink in Wright's stain, giving the cytoplasm a stippled appearance. ($\times$1,160)

Figure 2. Electron micrograph of neutrophil. In this cell, the nucleus (N) is bilobed. A few large azurophilic granules (A) are dispersed among the smaller, less dense specific granules (SG). A Golgi complex (G) occupies the cell center. The cell membrane is irregular. Small pseudopodia are extended from its surface and some vacuoles (V) are produced by the fusion of pseudopodia. ($\times$11,400)

Figure 3. Electron micrograph of neutrophil. This mature cell contains four nuclear lobes (N) connected by strands not seen in this section plane. A centriole (Ce) and Golgi complex (G) occupy the cell center (centrosome). Ribosomes are evenly distributed throughout the cell. Azurophilic granules (A) and specific granules are located in the peripheral cytoplasm. A few lipid (Li) inclusions and vesicles of varying size are present.

The mature segmented neutrophil is the "first cellular line of defense" in the body's acute inflammatory response, following shortly the "triple response" or wheal-and-flare phenomenon produced by histamine. The cells are phagocytic and ingest foreign materials to form phagolysosomes. Ingestion of invading bacteria may result in death of the bacteria or neutrophil or both, with lysis and formation of debris.

The peripheral-blood neutrophils are not capable of division but are replaced by immature forms from the marrow; hence, in any acute inflammation, a "shift to the left" or increase in percentage of immature neutrophils may occur with a total increase or leukocytosis. In a severe long-standing acute or recurrent infection, the numbers of neutrophils may approach those seen in the neoplastic proliferation of leukemia. This is appropriately called a leukemoid reaction. In this instance, metamyelocytes and, rarely, myelocytes can be found in the peripheral blood.

Judged by the number of nuclear lobes, the cell in this figure is an older neutrophil. The paucity of ingested materials indicates that this cell has not been involved in an intense reaction to foreign materials. ($\times$18,000)

PLATE 38

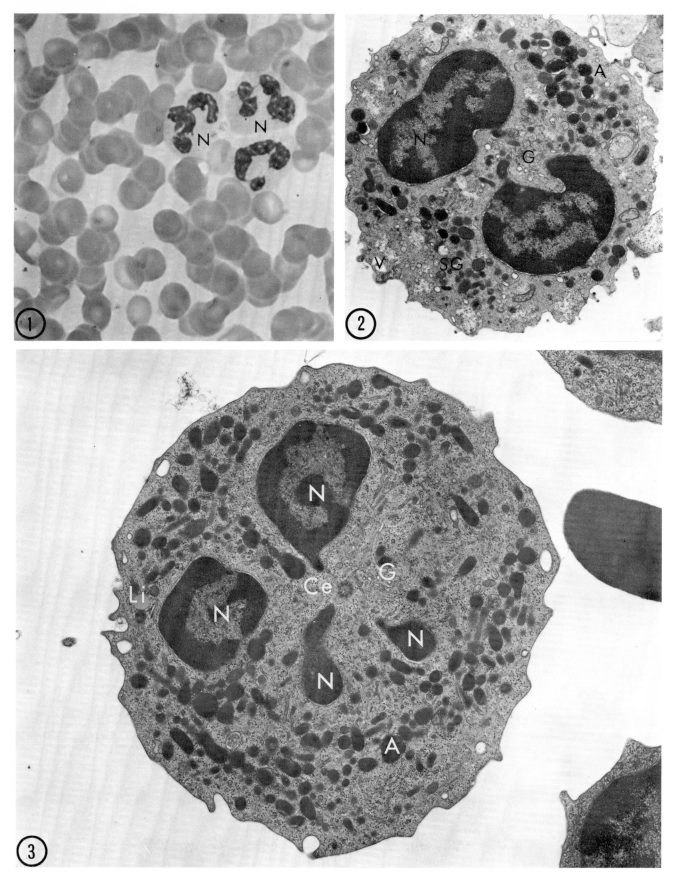

Plate 39 — GRANULOCYTE FORMATION

Figure 1. Photomicrograph of Wright's-stained marrow. Neutrophils, eosinophils, and basophils all follow the same sequence of development. In the normal adult, these cells develop in the marrow of long bones with megakaryocytes and erythrocytes, probably from a common hemocytoblast precursor. Lymphocytes and monocytes can develop here, but are produced largely in lymphoid tissues. In any marrow smear, different stages of formation of all cell types may be seen. In this view, a basophilic myelocyte (B), erythroblast (E), platelets (P), a neutrophil (N), and a promyelocyte (PM) may be recognized. As seen here, marrow smears contain many more nucleated cells per field than seen in peripheral blood smears. ($\times$1,160)

Figure 2. Electron micrograph of marrow. The sequence of formation of granulocytes begins with a myeloblast which differentiates into a promyelocyte (PM). Although similar to the myeloblast, this cell is characterized by the presence of large (0.5 to 1 μ) azurophilic granules (AG). Numerous free ribosomes (Ri) and mitochondria (M) are present. At this stage the ultimate type of granulocyte to be formed may be in doubt, as the cell-specific granules may not be present in the early stages. Subsequent formation of the specific granules (SG) makes identification certain. The adjacent more mature cell has specific granules typical of a neutrophil; this cell is a neutrophilic myelocyte. In addition to the presence of cell-specific granules, the overall cell size is smaller and the nucleus has a greater density in the myelocyte stage. Indentation of the nucleus, further reduction in size, and additional granules characterize the metamyelocyte stage. Granulocytes enter the circulation by diapedesis between narrow sinusoidal cells, usually at the "band" stage as lobulation of the nucleus begins. ($\times$6,200)

Figure 3. Electron micrograph of myeloblast. The myeloblast is a large pale-staining pluripotential cell. This cell can differentiate into promyelocytes, erythroblasts, or megakaryocytes. It has a large, finely granular nucleus (N). Few chromatin clumps are seen. The cytoplasm has scattered mitochondria, a small Golgi complex (G) and many free ribosomes (Ri). Some rough-surfaced endoplasmic reticulum (ER) is present. Several platelets (P) surround the myeloblast. ($\times$17,000)

84

PLATE 39

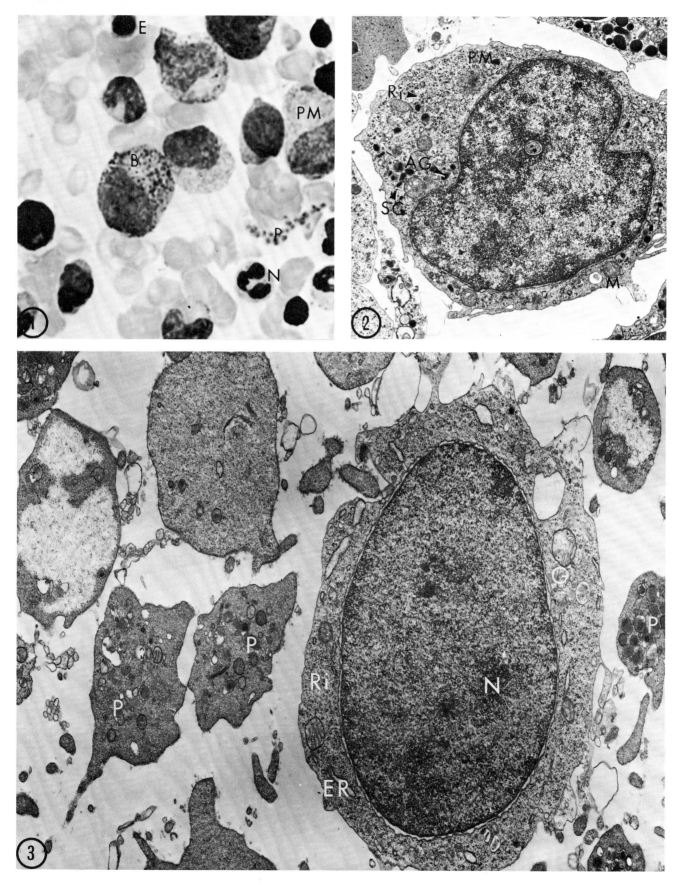

Plate 40 — EOSINOPHIL

Figure 1.   Photomicrograph of Wright's-stained eosinophil from peripheral blood smear. Eosinophils number approximately 1 to 3% of the leukocytes in peripheral blood, ranging from 50 to 300 cells per mm³ of blood. They are slightly larger than neutrophils, with diameters of 10 to 15 μ. These cells usually have a bilobed nucleus (N) obscured by numerous large acidophilic granules. ($\times$3,400)

Figure 2.   Electron micrograph of eosinophilic myelocyte. Young eosinophils have a single nucleus showing no indentation, a Golgi complex, and several specific granules in the cytoplasm in different states of maturation. Immature granules (FG) are limited by a membrane and contain a granular material. Mature specific granules (SG) are larger and contain a central dense homogeneous material surrounded by the granular substance seen in the forming granules. ($\times$18,500)

Figure 3.   Electron micrograph of mature eosinophil. The nucleus (N) is bilobed; the lobes are connected by a narrow strand of karyoplasm out of the plane of section. A large Golgi complex (G) occupies the cell center. The rounded or oval specific granules (SG) are about 0.5 to 1.5 μ in diameter; they are limited by an outer membrane. These granules contain protein crystalline structures with surrounding lipoid material. Specific granules in some mammals are ordered so that the central crystalline protein and the surrounding granular substance resemble a hamburger viewed from the edge. This ordered arrangement of the two components is not often seen in human eosinophil granules. A few azurophilic granules may be found. The granules may contain histamine and other "pressor amines." These cells have been associated with allergic phenomena, parasitic infections and stress reactions, as might be expected from their granule content. They are poor phagocytes but are associated with generalized lysosomal activity in subacute inflammatory processes. Administration of hydrocortisone markedly decreases the number of eosinophils in peripheral blood. ($\times$12,500)

86

PLATE 40

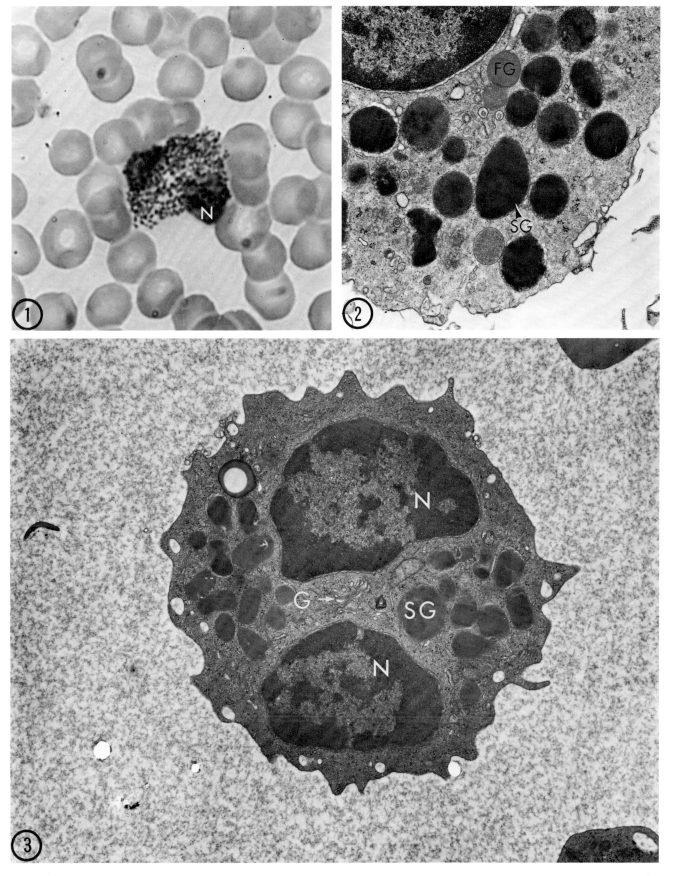

Plate 41 — BASOPHIL

Figure 1.   Photomicrograph of Wright's-stained blood smear. Basophils (B) are the least numerous leukocytes, comprising approximately 0.5% of the leukocytes and ranging from 25 to 50 cells per mm^3. Half of the volume of the basophil is occupied by its nucleus, which is usually irregular in shape and may be segmented. It is usually masked by dense basophilic cytoplasmic granules. The cell contains several metachromatic granules similar to those of mast cells, indicating a possible heparin component. These granules are usually ovoid but may show clumping. Erythrocytes (E) and a portion of a neutrophil (N) are also included in the field. ($\times$2,600)

Figure 2.   Electron micrograph of basophil. The nucleus of the basophil may be indented, elongated, or S shaped as seen here. The cytoplasm contains few organelles. Specific granules (SG) of basophils are water soluble and may disappear following routine fixative procedures, leaving empty rounded vacuoles. ($\times$13,000)

Figure 3.   Electron micrograph of basophil. In this cell, the integrity of the specific granules (SG) has been retained. The fine structure of the granules varies; it has been described as homogeneous, although a lamellar component has been seen in some granules. The granules in this basophil are irregular in shape and limited by an outer membrane; they show an electron-dense component associated with a finely granular matrix. Basophils may contain 50% of the blood histamine presumably a part of the specific granules. The nucleus (N) of this cell is small and is not electron dense. Mitochondria (M) and a small Golgi complex are interspersed between the specific granules. ($\times$26,000)

PLATE 41

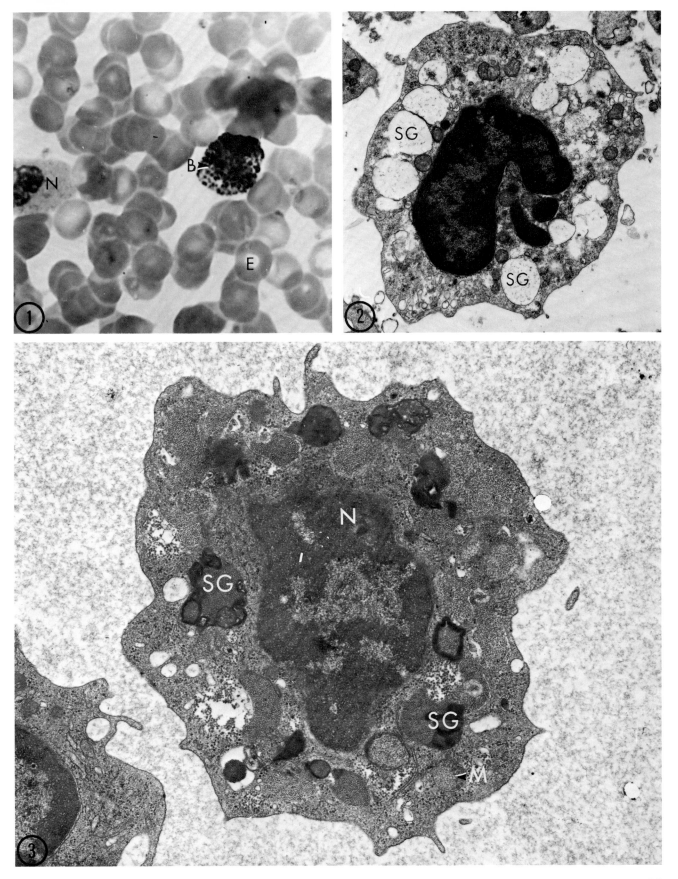

Plate 42 – MONOCYTE

Figure 1. Photomicrograph of Wright's-stained monocyte. Monocytes (M) comprise 3 to 10% of normal blood leukocytes. They are usually larger than other leukocytes, ranging from 12 to 15 μ in diameter. The nucleus may be ovoid or indented and may appear folded. It is not as basophilic as a lymphocyte nucleus, and the cytoplasm of monocytes is more abundant than that of lymphocytes. A neutrophil (N) lies next to the monocyte in this figure. The surrounding erythrocytes give a ready means of size determination. (×900)

Figure 2. Electron micrograph of monocyte. The nucleus (N) is both horseshoe shaped and indented. The cell center is occupied by a Golgi complex (G) and mitochondria. A few azurophilic granules (AG) accumulate in the peripheral cytoplasm. (×10,500)

Figure 3. Electron micrograph of monocyte. The nucleus (N) is horseshoe shaped. No nucleoli are included in this plane of section but a few nucleoli are present. Vesicles of the Golgi complex (G) and some mitochondria can be seen in the concavity of the nucleus. This cell center also contains centrioles (Ce). Some rough-surfaced endoplasmic reticulum (ER), azurophilic granules, lysosomes (Ly) and free ribosomes are located in the peripheral cytoplasm. The cell border is irregular and has several small processes. Monocytes develop in myeloid and lymphoid regions and become tissue macrophages after they leave the general circulation by diapedesis. (×16,400)

PLATE 42

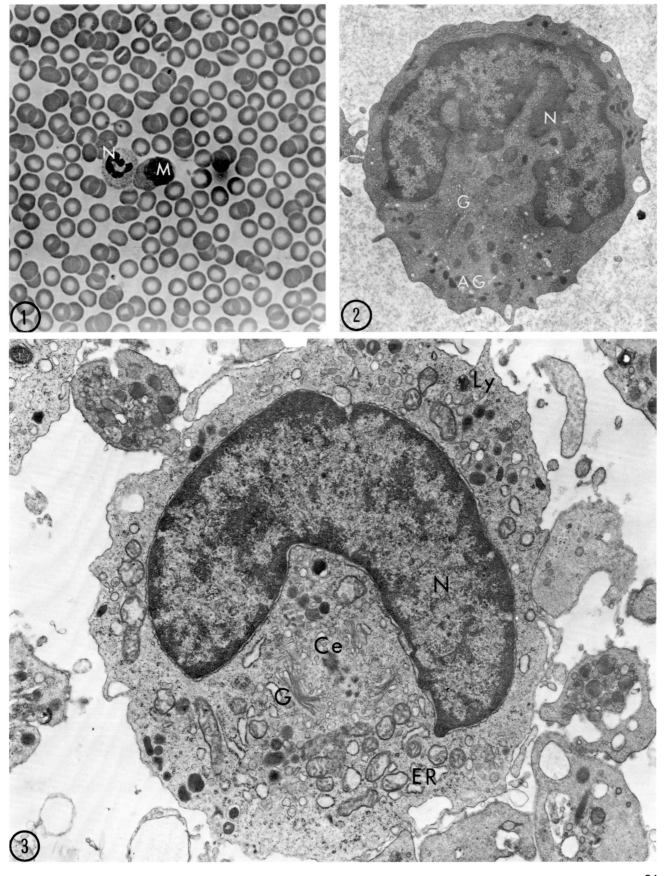

Plate 43 — LYMPHOCYTE

Figure 1. Photomicrograph of lymphocytes (Ly) in Wright's-stained blood smear. The nucleus is dense, intensely basophilic, round, and slightly eccentric. The cytoplasm is sparse. Lymphocytes are agranulocytes contributing 25 to 33% of circulating leukocytes, ranging from 1,500 to 3,000 per mm^3. Their size varies; the most numerous have diameters of 6 to 9 μ although larger ones, attaining a diameter of 25 μ, have been described. Erythrocytes are seen in the field and give a ready means of size comparison. ($\times$700)

Figure 2. Electron micrograph of lymphocyte. Lymphocytes have a round or indented nucleus (N) which is electron dense due to the presence of large amounts of heterochromatin. Chromatin clumps are large and often are apposed against the nuclear membrane, giving a "halo" effect. Nucleoli may be seen in electron micrographs, but one was not located in this plane of section. The nucleoli are poorly distinguished with the light microscope. Lymphocytes have a scanty cytoplasm. Several small pseudopodia (Ps) are seen at the periphery. Occasionally one of these pseudopods becomes enlarged at one end and is called a uropod. Microspikes and pinocytotic vesicles often form on the uropod, giving the lymphocyte an ameboid capacity. Free ribosomes are distributed in the cytoplasm. Parts of three platelets are seen at the corners of the figure. ($\times$14,000)

Figure 3. Electron micrograph of lymphocyte. This large lymphocyte has been called a prolymphocyte by some investigators. The nucleus (N) is slightly indented and contains peripherally condensed heterochromatin. These lymphocytes have the capacity to divide, and many serve as a reservoir of immunologically "uncommitted" cells. The cytoplasm contains an abundance of free ribosomes (R). Mitochondria (M) are tubular, contain several cristae and are more abundant on one pole of the cell. Centrioles (Ce) and a Golgi complex (G) are also seen at the cell pole. A few pseudopodia are extended from the cell border. Azurophilic granules may be seen in approximately 10% of lymphocytes but none is seen in this cell. ($\times$22,000)

PLATE 43

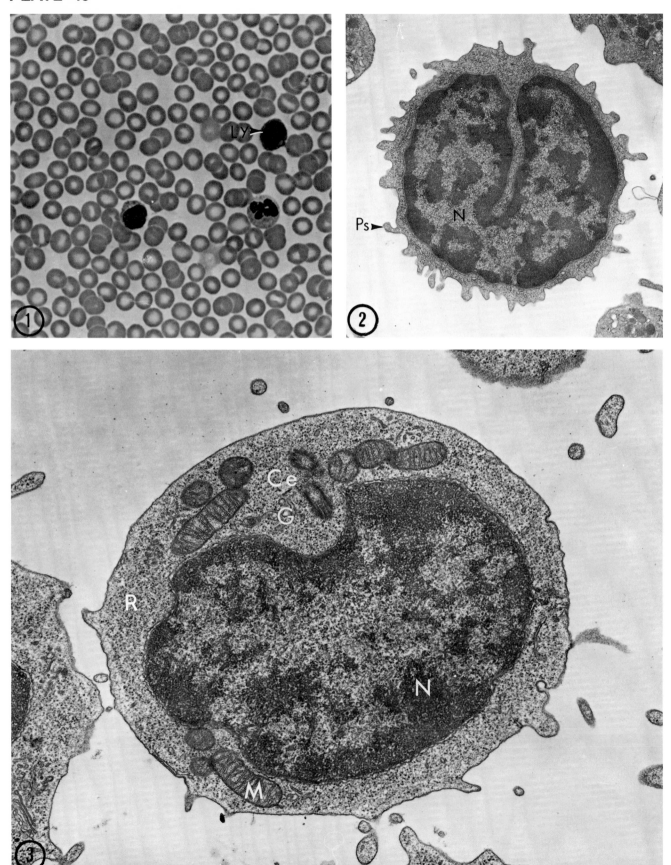

Plate 44 – LYMPHOCYTE FORMATION

Figure 1.   Photomicrograph of lymph nodule. Lymphocytes are formed in structures within lymphoid organs called lymph nodules. Nodules consist of clusters of lymphocytes supported by a reticular fiber stroma. The central portion of the nodule consists of larger, lighter-staining, more primitive cells: the lymphoblasts, plasmablasts, and possibly monoblasts. This lighter-staining region is the germinal center (GC). Arterioles (A) often serve as structures around which the nodules are formed. Lighter-staining reticular cells are interspersed between the lymphocytes. ($\times$150)

Figure 2.   Electron micrograph of young lymphocyte in germinal center. Lymphoblasts and young lymphocytes have more cytoplasm and often have tubular processes (P). Mitochondria are small and are usually round or oval. The cytoplasm is filled with free ribosomes (Ri). ($\times$25,000)

Figure 3.   Electron micrograph of lymph nodule. Lymphocytes (L) in different stages of maturation are arranged in tight clusters. The lymphocytes are separated by fine reticular fibers and processes of reticular cells (P). The reticular cells (Re) are larger than the lymphoid elements, and have more cytoplasm and a larger nucleus. Mitochondria, free ribosomes and a few tubules of rough-surfaced endoplasmic reticulum are present but sparse. ($\times$8,600)

PLATE 44

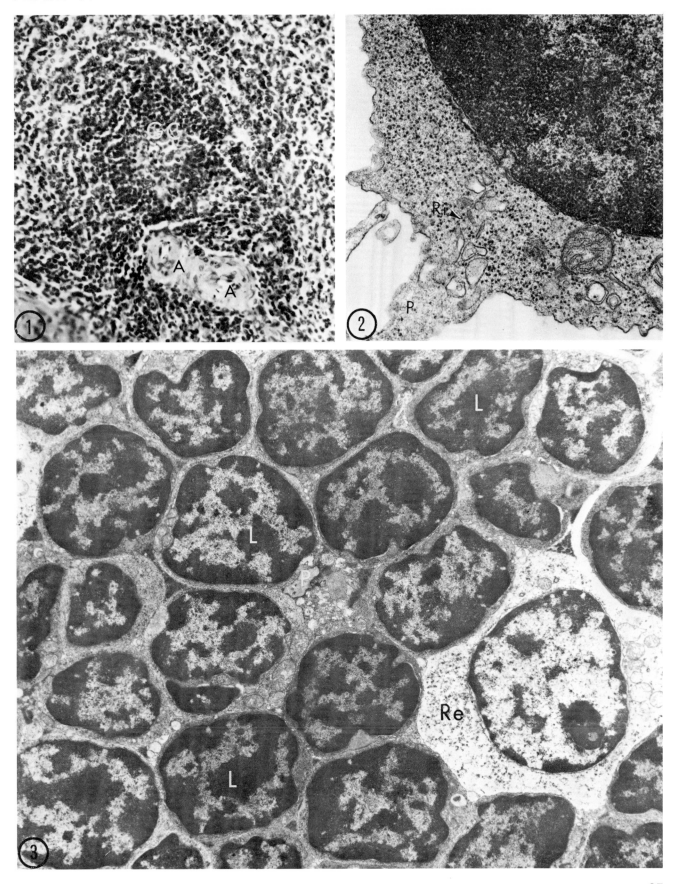

95

Plate 45 — PLATELET

Figure 1. Photomicrograph of marrow smear. Aggregates of platelets (P) appear as clumped masses of granular structures on dried films. Leukocytes (L) and a megakaryocyte (M) in the field may be used to compare with the size of individual platelets. Platelets are membrane-bound bodies of cytoplasm without nuclear material. They range from 2 to 4 μ in diameter, depending on whether they are floating free or are spread out on a film. They average 300,000 platelets per mm³ in normal subjects. In slide preparations, platelets often form clumps because of their specific capacity to agglutinate. The platelet shows a clear cytoplasm (hyalomere) with a granular center (the granulomere). ($\times$580)

Figure 2. Electron micrograph of platelet. Since the platelet is a fragment of cytoplasm of a megakaryocyte, it may contain organelles or inclusions of the mother cell. In this platelet, a centriole (Ce), mitochondria (M) and specific granules (SG) were trapped. The latter two structures are characteristic of all platelets. The plasma membrane (PM) has a thin plasma-protein and mucopolysaccharide film adhering to its outer surface. ($\times$4,000)

Figure 3. Electron micrograph of platelet. The characteristic granules of the chromatomere (Ch) are randomly distributed in the homogeneous hyalomere (Hy). Elements of microtubules, mitochondria (M), microfilaments and parts of Golgi vesicles are present in the hyalomere. The chromatomere consists of a group of membrane-limited round granules (0.2 to 0.3 μ) containing a granular substance. These are called A granules or alpha granulomeres, and are thought to have lysosomal properties. These granules may contain serotonin and other kinins important in postcapillary vessel contraction and control of hemorrhage.

Other granules ("very dense granules") have been described for some platelets but are rare in human platelets. Platelet agglutination is stimulated by many factors. Contact with collagen or adenosine diphosphate (ADP) may cause platelet-platelet interaction. Ultrastructural changes which follow stimulation are: central grouping of organelles and formation of numerous pseudopods (Ps); agglutination; thrombocytorrhexis (disruption of the A granules and of the platelet plasma membrane (PM), particularly in the center of a platelet cluster, or thrombus). These events are followed by thrombocytolysis with general disintegration of the entire thrombus. ($\times$32,000)

Figure 4.
Insert. Electron micrograph of fibrin. Platelet lysis releases platelet factor 3 which functions in thromboplastin formation and causes thrombin formation, a substance critical to conversion of soluble fibrinogen to insoluble fibrin. Fibrin appearance is similar to that of collagen strands, but shows an axial periodicity of about 25 mμ, less than half the periodicity of collagen. Plasma-soluble fibrinogen is composed of three pairs of chains: two A, two B, and two C chains having different active terminal groups. Thrombin causes cleavage of the fibrinogen forming the fibrin monomer. This molecule is longer than the fibrin periodicity so polymerization must involve an orderly overlapping of monomer units. ($\times$54,000)

96

PLATE 45

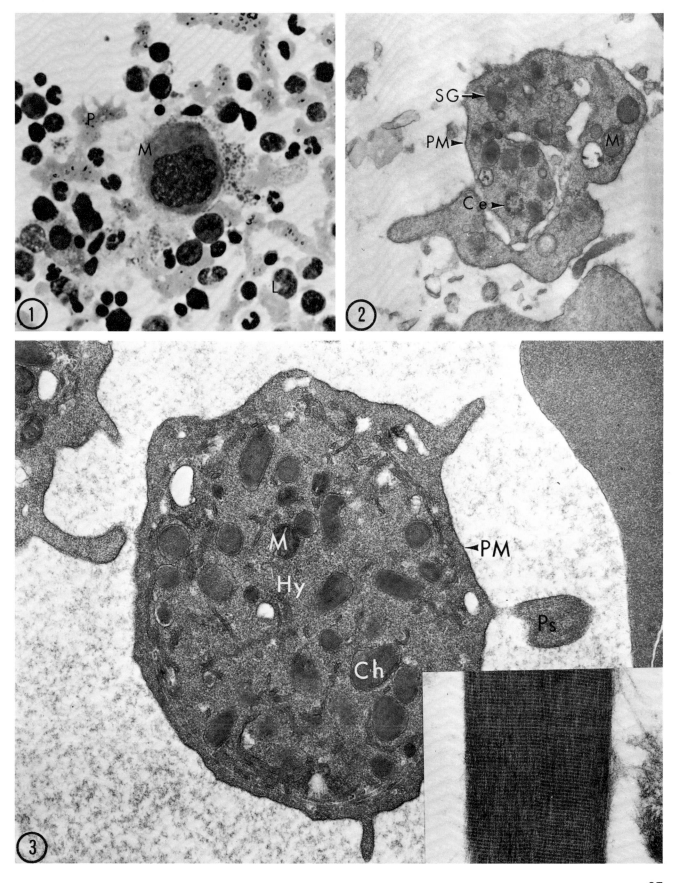

Plate 46 — MEGAKARYOCYTE

Figure 1.   Photomicrograph of Wright's-stained marrow smear. Myeloblasts form mega-karyocytes as well as the erythroid and granulocyte series. Megakaryocytes form platelets. Megakaryocytes (Mk) are huge cells (30 to 150 μ) with large multilobed nuclei. Thin strands of karyoplasm connect the large lobes. The cytoplasm is finely granular and generally basophilic. The cell surface is irregular, with many cytoplasmic pseudopods. ($\times$600)

Figure 2.   Photomicrograph of epon-embedded section of marrow. Large lipid droplets (L) and elements of myeloid tissue surround a giant megakaryocyte (Mk). The nucleus is lobed and contains several nucleoli. The cytoplasm hyalomere is filled with small granules (the chromatomere). Platelets are often seen at the periphery of these cells. ($\times$650)

Figure 3.   Electron micrograph of part of one megakaryocyte. Small electron-dense gran-ules (arrows) occupy the hyalomere part of the cytoplasm. These acidophilic granules are about 100 mμ in diameter and are the same as the alpha granules of platelets. The cytoplasm of the megakaryocyte is divided peripherally into regions the size of platelets by a complex infolding of the cell membrane. This often resembles a canalicular system of membrane vesicles (V) within the cell, and finally develops into a true segmentation of megakaryocyte cytoplasm. Most organelles, mitochondria, Golgi complex and rough-surfaced endoplasmic reticulum (ER) are in the central region of the cytoplasm, although about three mitochondria with two to three cristae are seen in each cleavage field. Platelets form by separating at these cleavage planes. The nuclear lobes (NL) are con-nected by narrow strands of karyoplasm (NS). Nucleoli (Nu) are prominent. ($\times$5,000)

PLATE 46

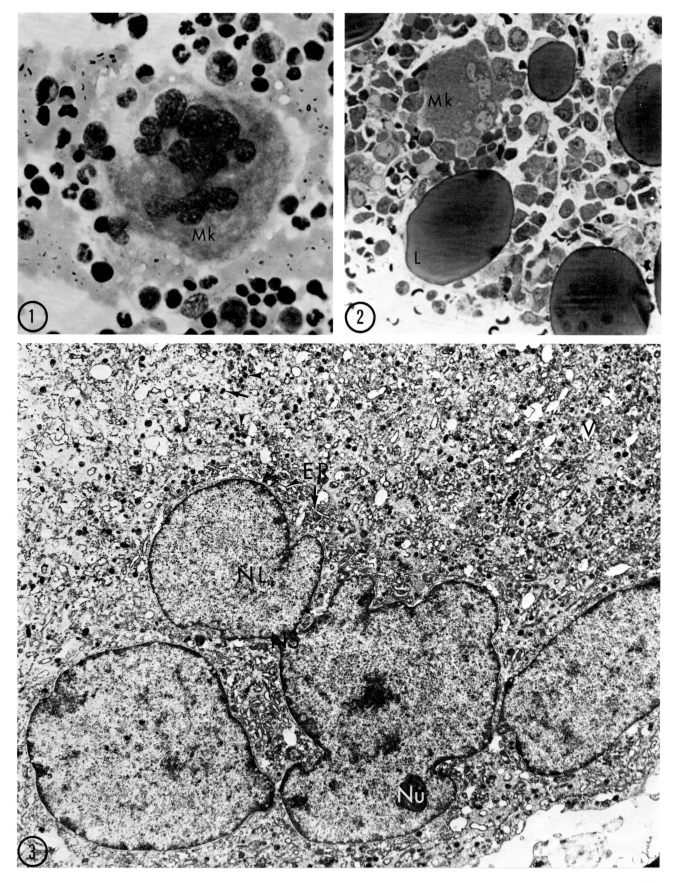

Muscle

PLATE 53

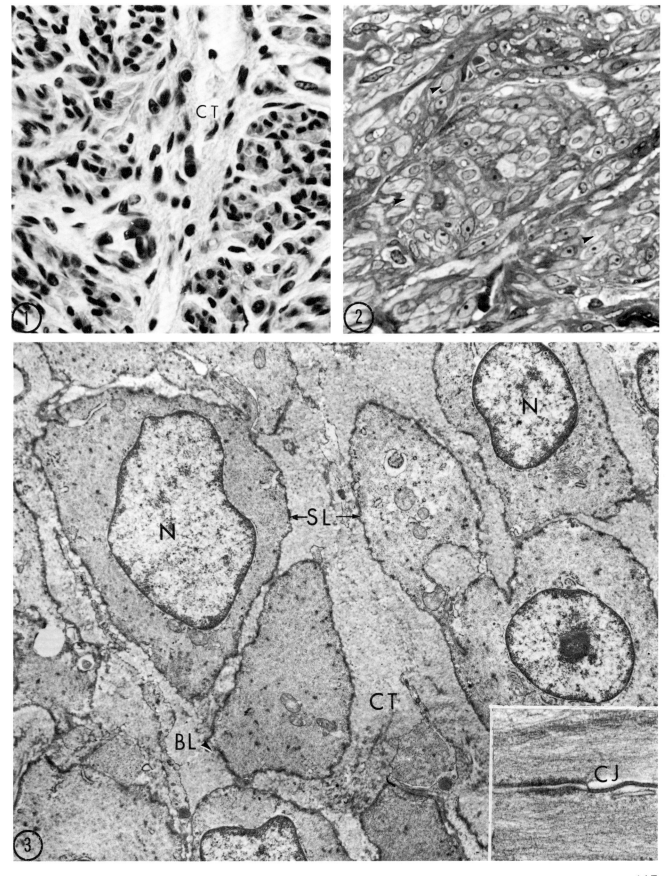

Plate 54 — CARDIAC MUSCLE

Figure 1.   Photomicrograph of longitudinal section of cardiac muscle. Numerous vessels (C) are located between the sheets of branching fibers (cells) which are elongate, nontapered structures. Each cell contains a pale, centrally placed ovoid nucleus. The darker nuclei are from either fibroblasts or endothelial cells. Lateral boundaries of the fibers are readily distinguished as they are separated by a loose fibrous endomysium. The cross-striated pattern of these cells is not seen as readily with hematoxylin-eosin (H&E) as is the striated pattern of skeletal muscle. Phosphotungstic acid hematoxylin (PTAH) staining enhances the cross-striated appearance. ($\times$375)

Figure 2.   Photomicrograph of epon-embedded cardiac muscle. In this thin section, the characteristic cross-striated pattern of the myofibrils can be seen. At the points of contact of adjacent cells, special junctions called intercalated discs (ID) appear as dark lines. These are most prominent at the ends of muscle fibers, but some discs may also follow the lateral boundary of cells for a short distance. ($\times$600)

Figure 3.   Electron micrograph of cardiac muscle fiber. The nucleus (N) of cardiac fibers is usually located near the center of the cell, but this nucleus is close to the sarcolemma (Sl). The nucleus appears as two because the section was made through a nuclear cleft. Myofibrils (Mf) are deposed longitudinally and show typical sarcomeres. Mitochondria (M) are concentrated in the perinuclear sarcoplasm and between myofibrils. A capillary (C) is close to the sarcolemma. Pinocytotic vesicles are numerous along the sarcolemma adjacent to the capillary. ($\times$6,800)

Figure 4.   Electron micrograph of intercalated disc. Intercalated discs (ID) consist of the plasma membranes of adjacent cells in close apposition but separated by a definitive intercellular space except at a few sites where the two membranes appear fused, as commonly seen at tight junctions (TJ). These small areas of direct contact may be significant in the contraction excitation of contiguous cells. The discs often appear to be continuous and extend beyond the junction of two abutted cells. A disc may follow a zigzag course across several muscle-fiber junctions. Since the ends of all fibers involved are not in register, intercalated junctions are formed along some lateral membrane sites in addition to the junctions at the ends. The disc at each cell is irregular and follows the staggered ends of myofibrils. Two kinds of junctions are seen at the disc: true desmosomes (D) with actin thin filaments serving the function of tonofibrils, and tight junctions (TJ) where the usual intercellular space of about 20 mμ is obliterated. ($\times$10,000)

116

PLATE 54

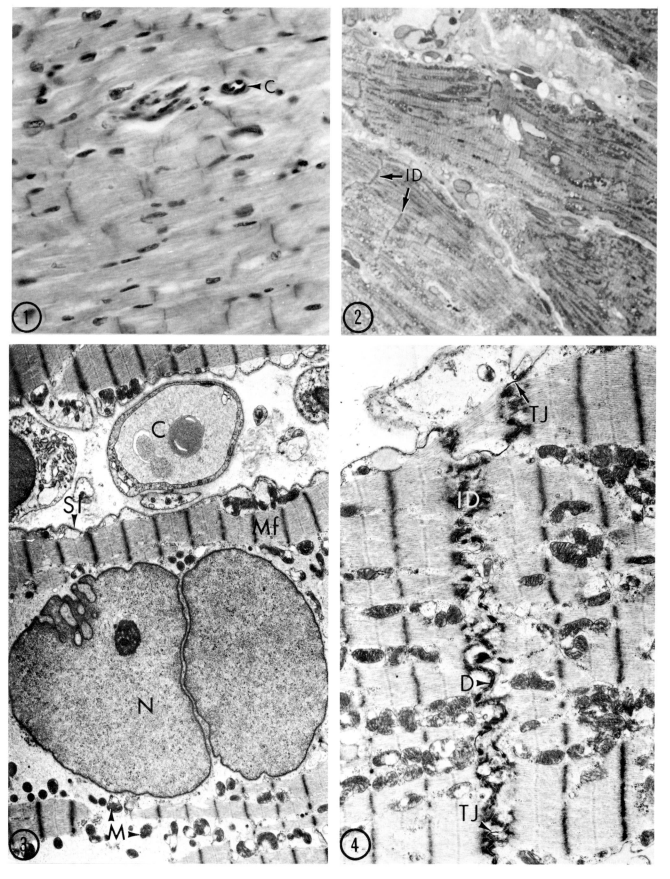

Plate 55 — CARDIAC MUSCLE

Figure 1.   Photomicrograph of cross section of cardiac muscle. Cross sections of cardiac muscle fibers (MF) show the nuclei (N) to be round structures centrally disposed in somewhat irregularly shaped fibers. Muscle fibers are grouped into fasicles separated by a connective-tissue perimysium, capillaries, and some fibers of autonomic nerves. (×200)

Figure 2.   Photomicrograph of epon-embedded cross section of cardiac muscle. Each muscle fiber contains an oval light-staining nucleus (N) with a nucleolus. Nuclei may be eccentric but are rarely peripherally positioned. Alternate wavy light and dark bands within the cytoplasm are a function of oblique sectioning of the myofibrils. The fibers are surrounded by a fibrous endomysium supporting several capillaries (C). (×600)

Figure 3.   Electron micrograph of cardiac muscle fiber. Cardiac muscle has the same cross-striation pattern seen in voluntary muscle. Longitudinally placed myofibrils (Mf) are separated by mitochondria (M) and tubules of sarcoplasmic reticulum (SR). These tubules are not as extensive as those in voluntary muscle. Larger mitochondria are found in the cytoplasm just inside the sarcolemma (Sl). Pinocytotic vesicles (PV) are seen at the sarcolemma, which is surrounded by a thin basal lamina in which collagen fibrils of the endomysium (E) are buried. A capillary (C) lies close to the muscle fibers. This partially contracted muscle fiber shows accordion-like folds of sarcolemma (Sl) with the sarcolemma remaining close to the myofibrils at their Z lines (Z). The longitudinally disposed myofilament arrangement is highly ordered, resulting in the cross-striated pattern of the myofibrils. This arrangement is described in more detail in Plate 49. Special cell junctions unique to cardiac muscle are the intercalated discs shown in Plate 54. (×16,000)

PLATE 55

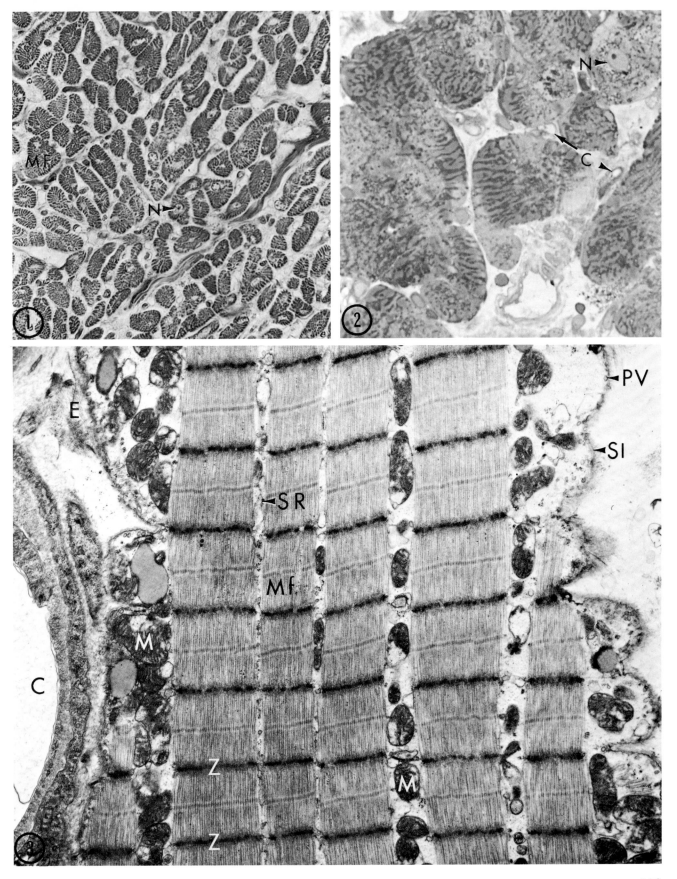

Nerve

Plate 56 — PERIPHERAL NERVE: NODE OF RANVIER

Figure 1. Photomicrograph of peripheral nerve. Nerves consist of groups of nerve fibers (NF) surrounded and supported by connective tissue. Each nerve fiber is invested in cytoplasmic folds of Schwann cells the nuclei (N) of which are interspersed among the nerve fibers. Large fibers have myelin sheaths formed by the investing membranes of the Schwann cells. The myelin and the Schwann cells are the neurilemma. The nerve fibers appear wavy and usually stain less intensely than the surrounding tissue. In this preparation, the tissue was post-fixed in osmium that stained the myelin sheath and surrounding lipid (L) in the connective tissue. Ordinary histologic stains do not dye the myelin sheaths, leaving a halo around each nerve fiber. (×370)

Figure 2. Photomicrograph of peripheral nerve. The tissue in this figure was post-fixed in osmium that stained the myelin sheath (MS) black. Collagen fibers of the endoneurium (En) separate adjacent nerve fibers (NF). The myelin sheath is interrupted periodically where adjacent Schwann cells of the neurilemma meet along the fiber axis. These sites of Schwann-cell junctions are the nodes of Ranvier (NR). Myelin is absent at these junctions. (×600)

Figure 3. Electron micrograph of node of Ranvier. Axis cylinders (AC) are invested by Schwann cells (SC). As axis cylinders are usually longer than their investing cells, several Schwann cells form the sheath of peripheral nerve fibers with each Schwann cell investing one segment of axis cylinder. Areas at the union of successive Schwann cells constitute nodal areas where areas of invested axis cylinders are the internode regions. As shown in the cross section of peripheral nerve (Plate 57), the myelin sheath results from successive layering of Schwann-cell plasma membranes. In this view, the myelin sheath (MS) terminates on either side of the node (N). Cytoplasmic processes (P) of the Schwann cells occupy the nodal region devoid of myelin. In cross section, inner and outer mesaxons representing the leading edge of the folding Schwann-cell membranes are seen. In longitudinal section, the cytoplasm between Schwann-cell membrane folds (MF) becomes prominent on the axolemma surface as the myelin sheath terminates at the node. The axon contains neurofilaments (Nf), microtubules (Mt) and elongated mitochondria (M). The axis cylinder and Schwann cells are surrounded by a thin basal lamina (BL) continuous across the node. Outside the basal lamina, collagen (Co) fibers of the endoneurium separate and support individual nerve fibers. A Schwann-cell process is also included in the field. (×21,000)

122

PLATE 56

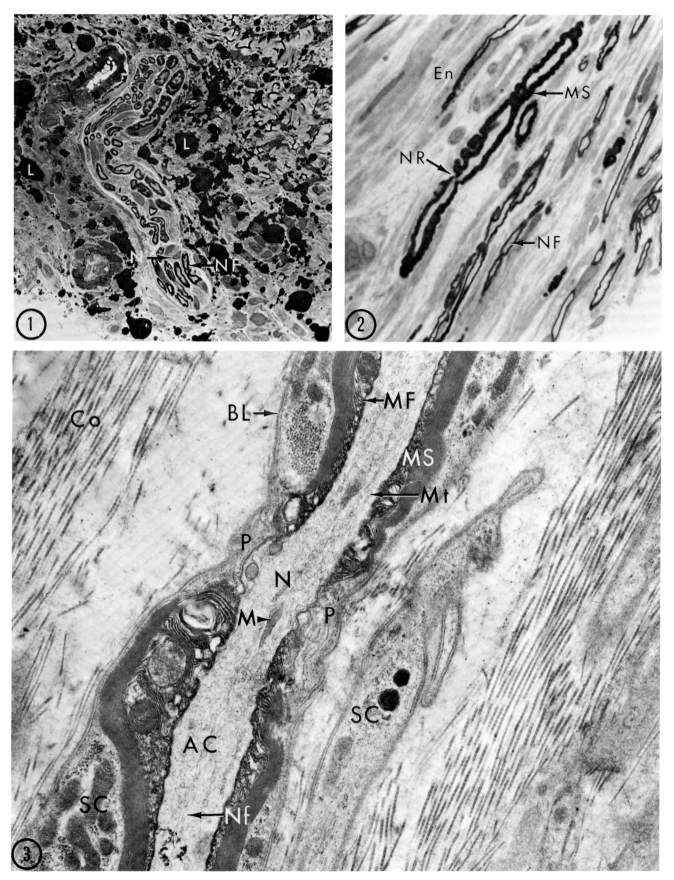

Plate 57 — PERIPHERAL NERVE: CROSS SECTION

Figure 1. Photomicrograph of peripheral nerve, H&E stain. In sections stained with ordinary dyes such as H&E, isolated axons in groups of nerve fibers are difficult to delineate; the axis cylinders and the neurilemma stain poorly. However, Schwann-cell and fibroblast nuclei (N) stain readily, so that the entire nerve is readily identified. In longitudinal and oblique sectioned nerves, the axons appear to follow a wavy course. The connective tissue surrounding a peripheral nerve is called the epineurium (E). Large nerves are compartmentalized by septa, the perineurium. Each axon has a connective-tissue sheath, the endo-neurium, accounting for the presence of fibroblasts within nerves. ($\times$150)

Figure 2. Photomicrograph of epon-embedded peripheral nerve. With special stains the myelin sheaths of large axons are readily shown. These appear in cross section as dark circles of varying sizes surrounded by fibroblasts. Schwann-cell nuclei are also seen. The axis cylinders within the myelin sheaths stain poorly. A connective-tissue sheath, the epineurium (En) surrounds the nerve. Arterioles (A), a venule (V) and capillaries (C) are also seen in the surrounding connective tissue. ($\times$150)

Figure 3. Electron micrograph of unmyelinated nerve. All peripheral nerve fibers are ensheathed by Schwann cells (SC). In nonmyelinated fibers, several axis cylinders may be surrounded by cytoplasmic folds, mesaxons (Ma), of the same Schwann cell. The axis cylinders contain mitochondria (M) and neurofibrils (Nf). The axis cylinders and their investing Schwann cells are surrounded by a thin basal lamina (BL) separating them from the surrounding collagenous connective tissue (CT). ($\times$26,000)

Figure 4. Electron micrograph of myelin sheath. Large axis cylinders (AC) are invested in several layers of Schwann-cell membranes constituting the myelin sheath (MS). During development of the myelin sheath, the axis cylinder is enfolded by the Schwann cell. The axolemma contacts the enfolded plasma membrane of the Schwann cell except at the outer surface, where the Schwann-cell membranes fail to close completely around the axis cylinder. The free margin of Schwann-cell membranes investing the axolemma is called a mesaxon. The wrapping of Schwann-cell cytoplasm continues to form a spiral of flattened membranes around the axis cylinder. The cytoplasm between opposing folds of SC membranes is extruded peripherally to the Schwann-cell body at the periphery of the forming sheath. These investing plasma membranes fuse forming a laminated structure consisting of alternating dark (D) and light (L) bands which repeat every 11 to 16 mμ. Occasionally, a fine band may bisect the light band; this represents fusion of the outer leaflets of the Schwann-cell membranes, limiting successive Schwann-cell processes. The dark bands are about 3 mμ thick and repeat every 12 mμ. The inner advancing SC process, the inner mesaxon (Ma), contacts the axolemma. The outer mesaxon (OMa) is seen at the upper left. ($\times$157,000)

124

PLATE 57

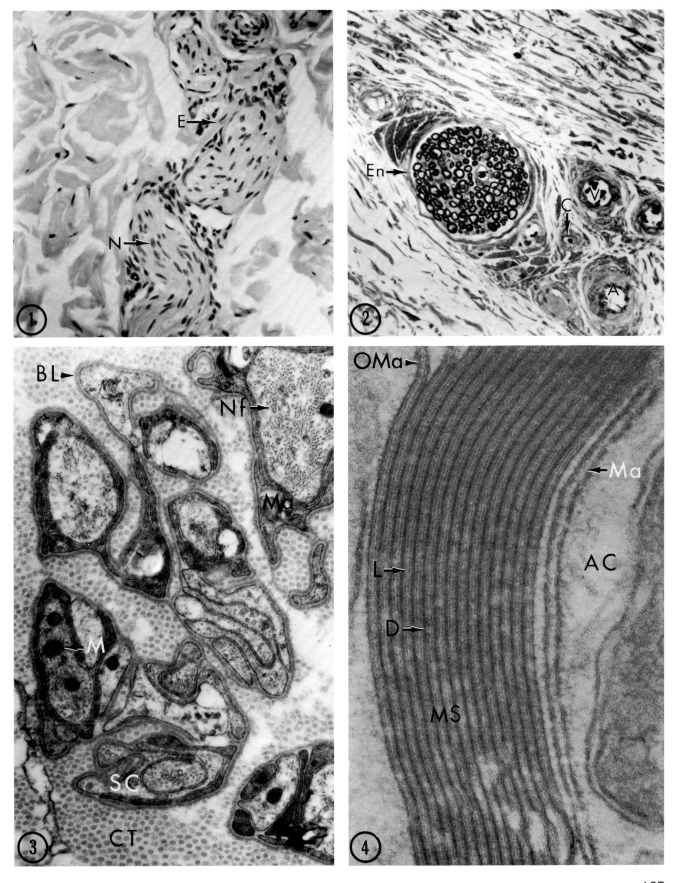

Plate 58 — SPINAL CORD

Figure 1.   Photomicrograph of a cross section of anterior horn of spinal cord. The spinal cord is ovoid in cross section as it is flattened anteroposteriorly. Neuron cell bodies and supporting glial cells constitute the gray matter in the center of the cord. Nerve fibers from these neurons course between these cells and move in both cephalic and caudal directions as they reach the surrounding white matter (WM). The gray matter is a column arranged so that an H shape is formed. The connecting bar of the H is the gray commissure connecting the two symmetrical halves of the column. The gray matter forms two dorsal horns and two anterior horns. The anterior horn (AH) shown here is broader and shorter than the posterior horn, and contains the largest neurons in the cord. These large neurons (N) are the anterior horn cells and give rise to the efferent fibers. Neurons of the posterior horns are smaller and receive afferent fibers. ($\times$65)

Figure 2.   Photomicrograph of anterior horn cell. The anterior horn cells (AHC) are the largest neurons in the cord; they are multipolar and contain many Nissl bodies (NB). Nissl bodies are present in the cytoplasm of the dendritic processes but do not occupy the cell axon. These cells have a large nucleus and a prominent nucleolus. Smaller neurons (N) are also present and serve as conduction bridges between neurons within the cord and neurons at other levels of the cord. Myelinated (M) and nonmyelinated fibers and neuroglia cells (Ng) constitute the surrounding neuropil. ($\times$375)

Figure 3.   Electron micrograph of anterior horn cell cytoplasm. The most prominent features of the cytoplasm of anterior horn cells and most neurons are the large basophilic bodies, the Nissl bodies (NB), groups of rough-surfaced vesicles and membranes separated by clusters of free ribosomes. In large neurons, as seen here, the rough-surfaced membranous vesicles are arranged almost parallel to adjacent membranous vesicles in the same Nissl body. This stacked arrangement is not found in smaller neurons, nor is the outline of individual Nissl bodies as distinct. Numerous small mitochondria (M), microtubules (Mt), and neurofilaments are dispersed between Nissl bodies. ($\times$6,500)

PLATE 58

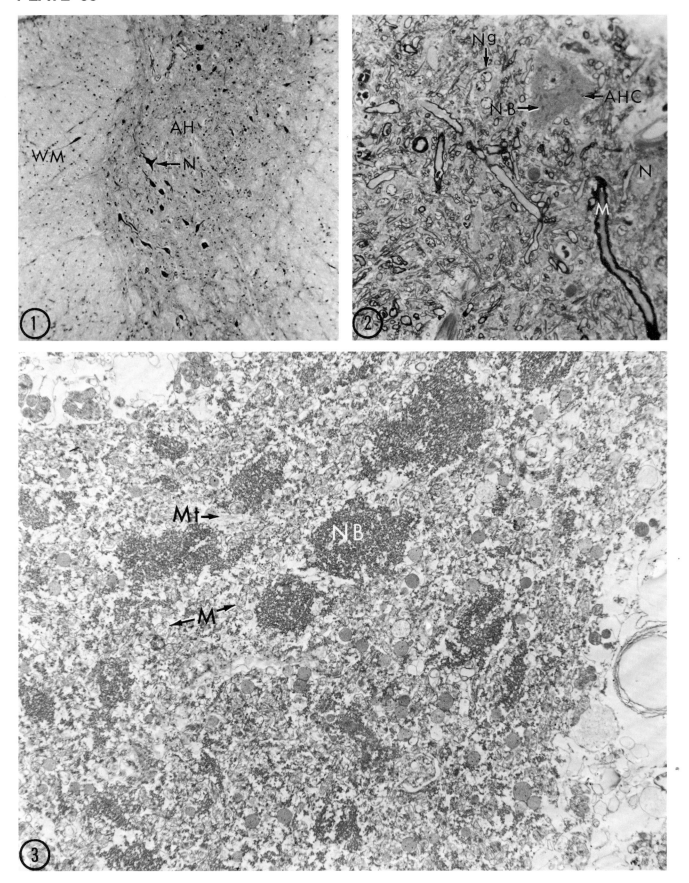

Plate 59 — CEREBRAL CORTEX

Figure 1. Photomicrograph of cerebral cortex. The cerebral cortex is a layer of gray matter covering the white matter of the cerebral hemispheres. The cortex generally shows six layers which vary in prominence in different cortical regions: molecular layer (most superficial), outer granular layer, pyramidal cell layer, inner granular layer, internal pyramidal layer and the layer of polymorphous cells. The huge pyramidal cells of the motor cortex are called Betz cells (BC). The cortical region between neurons is essentially structureless and consists of a poorly staining feltwork of naked nerve fibers and the processes of neuroglia cells. This is the neuropil (Np). Nuclei of the neuroglia cells (NC) are readily discerned. (×375)

Figure 2. Photomicrograph of epon-embedded section of cerebral cortex. Parts of two large neurons (Ne) are supported in the neuropil containing both myelinated (My) and nonmyelinated fibers (NF). The nuclei of the neurons are light staining because of the condensation of chromatin making the nucleolus very prominent. Small lipofuscin granules (Gr) occupy part of the cytoplasm. Neuroglia cells (NC) occur as satellites around the neurons. (×400)

Figure 3. Electron micrograph of neuron of cerebral cortex. The nucleus is light staining and contains several small electron-dense perichromatin granules that may represent the onset of a pathologic change. The cytoplasm contains widely distributed rough-surfaced endoplasmic reticulum (ER) surrounded by numerous free ribosomes, producing a dispersed Nissl-body pattern. Heterogeneous lipofuscin granules (LG) are randomly placed, as are the numerous mitochondria. Smooth-surfaced Golgi complexes (G) are also present. Neurofilaments are not prominent in this cell but are found in many neurons of the cerebral cortex. This neuron is surrounded by both myelinated and nonmyelinated axons and dendrites of the neuropil. (×14,300)

128

Circulatory System

Plate 66 – LARGE ARTERY

Figure 1.   Photomicrograph of large artery. Arteries consist of three walls: an inner tunica intima (TI), a tunica media (TM), and a tunica adventitia (TA). The tunica intima consists of an endothelial cell lining and its subjacent thin connective-tissue layer, the lamina propria. An elastic membrane, the internal elastic lamina (IEL), lies along the boundary between the intima and the muscular media. Other elastic laminae occur within the muscular layer in the largest arteries. External elastic laminae (EEL) lie between the media and the collagenous fibers of the tunica adventitia. (×375)

Figure 2.   Photomicrograph of distributing artery. Smaller arteries have the characteristic three walls but the number of elastic laminae is reduced. Elastic laminae are not seen in arterioles. In this vessel, the internal elastic lamina (IEL) bounds the media-intima interface. The muscle fibers (SM) of the tunica media are prominent but are not separated from the tunica adventitia (TA) by other elastic laminae. The lumen (Lu) of the vessel is slightly irregular due to loss of hydrostatic pressure and partial contraction with fixation. (×375)

Figure 3.   Electron micrograph of large artery. The endothelial cells lie upon a thin basal lamina (BL). The subjacent lamina propria consists of irregularly arranged collagen fibrils. Smooth muscle fibers (SM) of the tunica media are seen in both cross and oblique section. An irregular, wavy, electron-lucent elastic membrane, the internal elastic lamina (IEL), courses between the muscle fibers and the collagen fibrils of the lamina. The elastic lamina is interrupted by fenestrae. Although the elastic membrane is electron lucent, some internal fibrillar component (FC) can be distinguished. (×7,000)

Figure 4.   Electron micrograph of tunica intima of large artery. Smooth muscle (SM) fibers of the surrounding tunica media are surrounded by a thin basal membrane, and contain myofilaments and fusiform densities. The collagenous lamina propria (LP) of the tunica intima contains a fenestrated electron-lucent membrane, the internal elastic lamina (IEL). Endothelial cells line the vessel and extend small microvilli into the vessel lumen (L). (×7,000)

144

PLATE 66

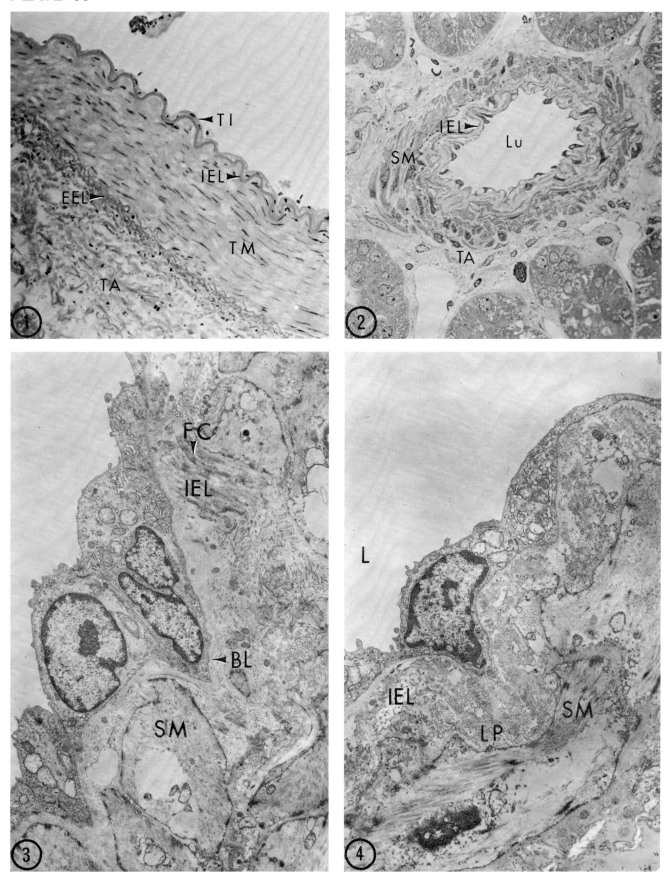

Plate 67 — VENULE

Figure 1. Photomicrograph of blood vessels in lamina propria. Blood vessels are distributed within a loose fibrous stroma. An arteriole (A) showing a thick muscular wall and a round lumen can be compared with the venule (V) which has a larger lumen and thinner walls. Smooth muscle constitutes most of the wall of the arteriole while a fibrous adventitia is prominent in the venule. Capillaries (C) are seen in cross section just below a larger thin-walled vein (V). ($\times$150)

Figure 2. Photomicrograph of epon-embedded venous sinus (VS). Erythrocytes fill the lumen. Simple squamous endothelial cells line the lumen, which is indented at the location of endothelial-cell nuclei. A collagenous adventitia and fibroblasts surround the endothelial cells. ($\times$375)

Figure 3. Electron micrograph of venule. Veins less than 100 μ in diameter are classed as venules. Simple squamous endothelial cells (EC) rest upon a basal lamina (BL). The nuclei (N) are elongated along the lumen (L) wall. The nucleus has finely condensed chromatin and contains a nucleolus (Nu). Small microvilli (Mv) and pinocytotic vesicles are present at the plasma membrane. A single row of smooth muscle cells or pericytes (P) is invested in the basal lamina. The nuclei of these cells are large but are not seen in this section. Their cytoplasm contains mitochondria and myofilaments. Collagen (Co) and fibroblasts (F) surround the muscles and comprise the tunica adventitia. Two erythrocytes (RBC) occupy the lumen. ($\times$7,000)

PLATE 67

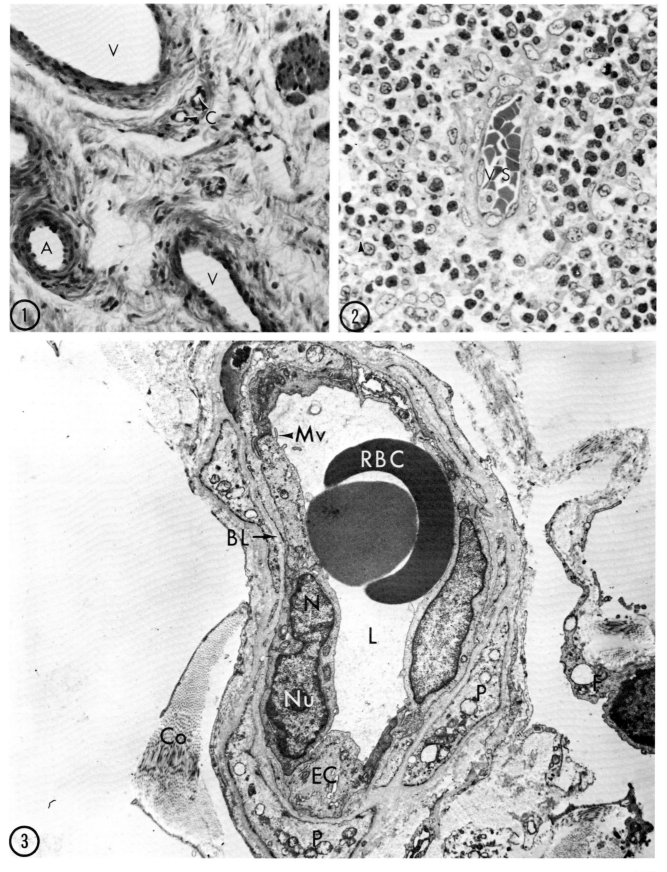

Plate 68 — SMALL ARTERY

Figure 1. Photomicrograph of cross section of artery. The endothelial cells lining the lumen (L) bulge into the lumen and appear close together because of the partial contraction of the vessel. The endothelial cells rest upon a basal lamina and are separated from the smooth muscle fibers (SM) of the tunica media by a thin elastic lamina. The tunica media is the most prominent layer, consisting of muscle fibers arranged in a circular direction. A thin layer of collagen and fibroblasts make up the tunica adventitia (TA), the fibers of which are anchored to the collagen in the adjacent connective tissue. In larger arteries, an elastic lamina is deposited between the tunica media and tunica adventitia. (×200)

Figure 2. Photomicrograph of epon-embedded blood vessels in connective tissue. The artery (A), seen here in longitudinal section, is thicker walled and has a smaller lumen than the adjacent vein (V). In this view, the smooth muscle fibers of the tunica media of the artery are seen in cross section. The nuclei are round in cross section and are centrally positioned. A layer of collagen fibers, the adventitia, surrounds the muscle. Small cross sections of a peripheral nerve (N) and a capillary (C) are above the artery. (×375)

Figure 3. Electron micrograph of cross section of arteriole. An erythrocyte (RBC) is in the lumen which is lined by simple squamous endothelial cells. These cells lie upon a basal lamina (BL). Adjacent endothelial cells meet and partially overlap. Tight junctions (TJ) anchor these junctions between the flattened edges of contiguous cells. The endothelial cells contain a nucleus (N) and mitochondria. Pinocytotic vesicles line the plasma membrane on both the luminal and basilar surfaces, and are also seen within the cell interior. These vesicles function in the transcellular movement of water and macromolecules. The tunica media consists of smooth muscle fibers arranged around the endothelium. Mitochondria are concentrated about the nucleus (N) of these fibers. The cytoplasm is filled with myofilaments. Fusiform dense structures are distributed among the filaments. A thin basal lamina surrounds each muscle fiber. Pinocytotic vesicles are also prominent on the sarcolemma. Collagen (Co) and fibroblasts (F) surround the muscle layer and make up the outer wall, the tunica adventitia. The fibroblasts extend thin processes around the vessel and follow the same direction taken by the muscle fibers. (×6,800)

PLATE 68

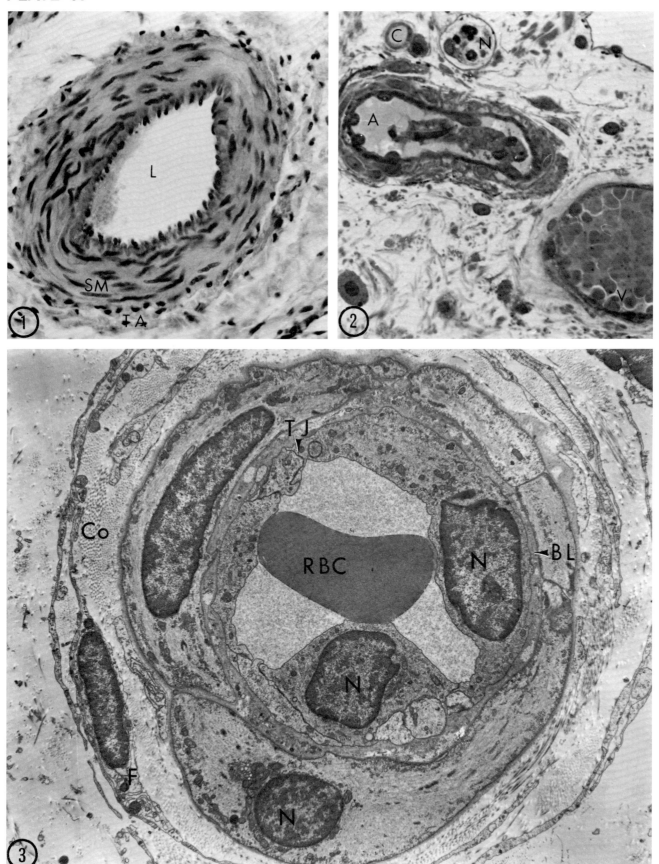

Plate 69 — CAPILLARY

Figure 1. Photomicrograph of capillary. Capillaries are the fundamental exchange unit of the vascular system. Plasma constituents and interstitial fluid are continuously exchanged across the capillary wall. To facilitate this movement of fluid and respiratory gases, the walls of capillaries are extremely thin and consist of the endothelial cell and a surrounding basal lamina. An erythrocyte is seen in the lumen of this large capillary (C). The diameters of capillaries vary from $20\,\mu$ to those which require distortion of the blood cells to squeeze through. Several veins (V) are present in the surrounding connective tissue. ($\times$600)

Figure 2. Electron micrograph of epon-embedded lymph nodule. Two capillaries (C) are seen in longitudinal section in this lymphocyte-rich field. Several erythrocytes are present in the lumen, which is narrow enough for the erythrocytes to contact the endothelial-cell walls. ($\times$375)

Figure 3. Electron micrograph of cross section of a capillary. Sections of cytoplasm of two simple squamous endothelial cells are united at their plasma membranes by tight junctions (TJ). Small lips of endothelial cells may project from these junctions into the lumen and are called marginal folds. Their cytoplasm contains mitochondria (M), free ribosomes (Ri), and some rough-surfaced endoplasmic reticulum (ER). Pinocytotic vesicles (PV) are present at the plasma membrane. A thin basal lamina (BL) contacts the thin outer surface. Some collagen is seen just outside the basal lamina. The cytoplasm of a pericyte partially surrounds the capillary. Pericytes are invested in a basal lamina and have several pinocytotic vesicles. The cytoplasm of these pericytes, unlike that of more differentiated smooth muscle fibers, does not contain myofilaments or fusiform densities in significant numbers. The pericytes (P) characteristically surround metarterioles, precapillaries and small venules. ($\times$25,000)

150

PLATE 69

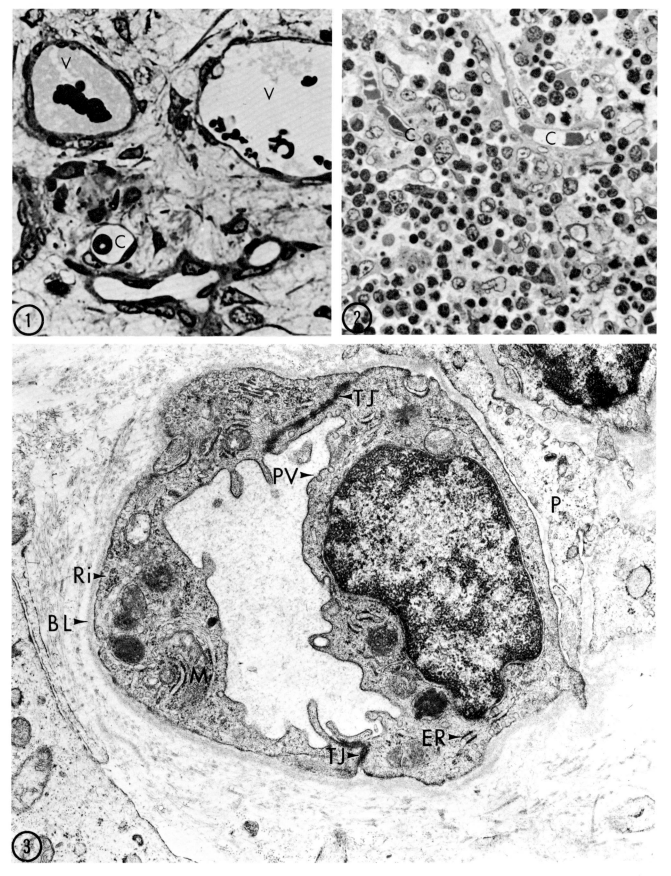

Lymphoid System

Plate 70 — LYMPH NODE

Figure 1.   Photomicrograph of cortex of lymph node. Lymph nodes are surrounded by a fibrous capsule (Ca) which extends trabeculae (T) into the node. A reticular network supports all of the cellular elements in a fibrillar mesh. The lymph node has a cellular cortical region and a less cellular medulla. The cortex consists of nodules (No) of lymphocytes containing a lighter-staining germinal center. The light staining is due to the presence of larger blast cells with more cytoplasm, resulting in greater distances between nuclei. The progeny of the blast cells migrate through the medulla and are collected in efferent lymph vessels at the hilus. Reticulocytes line the spaces through which the lymphoid cells emigrate. Lymph is brought to the lymph node by means of several afferent vessels (AV) which empty into the subcapsular space (SCS). Formed elements in the lymph also traverse the reticular mesh and exit via the efferent vessel and the medulla. (×150)

Figure 2.   Photomicrograph of epon-embedded lymph nodule. The lymph nodule consists of hundreds of lymphocytes and plasmacytes enmeshed in a reticular network. Reticulocytes (arrows) with larger lighter-staining nuclei are scattered between the lymphoid elements. The nodule has a rich supply of capillaries (C). A vein (V) is seen at the right of the figure. A small portion of germinal center (CG) is seen at the lower left. The cells of this region are large and have light-staining nuclei. (×375)

Figure 3.   Electron micrograph of germinal center of lymph nodule. Large cells with pale nuclei (N) are lymphoblasts. Numerous free ribosomes (Ri) and some mitochondria are found in the cytoplasm. This primitive cell is surrounded by cells with smaller and more granular nuclei (N) containing a prominent nucleolus (Nu). More organelles are found in these cells, which are fairly rich in ribosomes. A few reticular fibers (RF) separate the cells. Lymphocytes become immunologically competent and respond to antigens by becoming larger. These stimulated cells are pyroninophilic and contain many more ribosomes than the newly formed cells included in this figure. Monocytes may also be identified in lymph nodules; this raises the question of whether the large cells should be called lymphoblasts, monoblasts, plasmablasts, or hemocytoblasts. No morphologic distinction is made. (×9,200)

154

PLATE 70

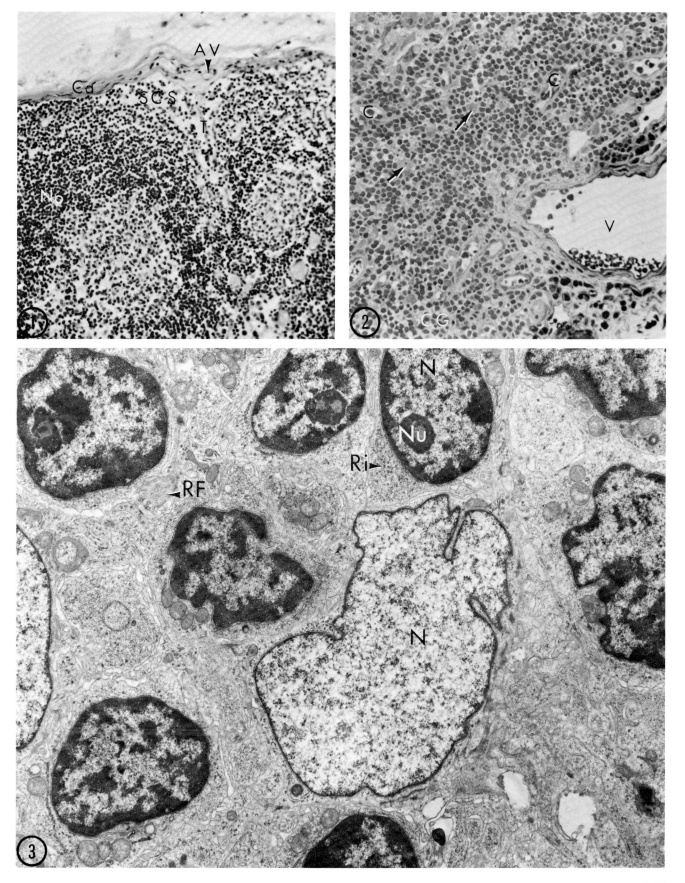

Plate 71 — SPLEEN

Figure 1. Photomicrograph of splenic corpuscle. The spleen is a lymphoid organ which circulates blood rather than lymph through its reticular spaces. It is encased in a fibroelastic capsule which may contain a few smooth muscle fibers. Trabeculae radiate into the spleen from the capsule and are accompanied by arteries. Branches of these trabecular arteries, the central arteries (CA), are eccentrically surrounded by clusters of basophilic lymphocytes forming splenic nodules (SN) which contain germinal centers. These nodules occur randomly throughout the substance of the spleen, in contrast to the peripheral distribution of nodules seen in lymph nodes. Two major areas are defined in the spleen: the white pulp (WP) and red pulp (RP). The former consists of the splenic nodules and the adjacent tissue into which the newly formed lymphoid cells are dispersed. The red pulp consists primarily of reticular cells and erythrocytes released in this area from a group of vessels branching from the central arteries. ($\times$140)

Figure 2. Photomicrograph of red pulp of spleen. The principal cells of the red pulp are the reticulocytes (R), which limit open spaces, and the sinusoids (S), occupied by erythrocytes and some leukocytes. A fine reticular network of basal lamellae surrounds the cell clusters, referred to as Billroth's cords. Venous sinuses (VS) receive blood from the sinusoids between the cords and are supported by an encircling layer of reticular fibers. Lining cells of the sinuses are oriented parallel to the vessel axis. ($\times$375)

Figure 3. Electron micrograph of red pulp. The circulation of blood through the red pulp has been extensively investigated. Two concepts have evolved. The open-circulation theory suggests that erythrocytes circulate freely between reticular cells ultimately entering the venous sinus. The closed theory suggests that erythrocytes are transported through a series of closed capillaries, ellipsoids, and sheathed vessels which empty directly into the venous sinuses. A compromise between these views seems correct from the arrangement seen in this figure. Reticulocytes (Re) line a sinusoidal space (S) occupied by erythrocytes (RBC) and leukocytes. Erythrocytes, platelets and leukocytes are also seen in the space on the other side of the basal lamina (BL). A flattened reticular cell (FRC) lies on one side of the basal lamina. The basal lamina is not a complete contiguous layer but is interrupted at intervals (arrow). These interruptions often occur at the point of union of adjacent reticular cells. Tight junctions (TJ) are present between some reticular-lining cells but the intercellular space of others appears to be approximated but patent, providing a means for transinusoidal movement of formed elements. The nuclei (N) of the reticular cells are granular, large and irregular. A nucleolus (Nu) is present. Mitochondria, lysosomes and rough-surfaced endoplasmic reticulum, as well as free ribosomes, are present. Pinocytotic vesicles are numerous on both sides of the cells. These cells are phagocytic and intact platelets, erythrocyte ghosts and disintegrating leukocytes may be found within them. ($\times$12,000)

PLATE 71

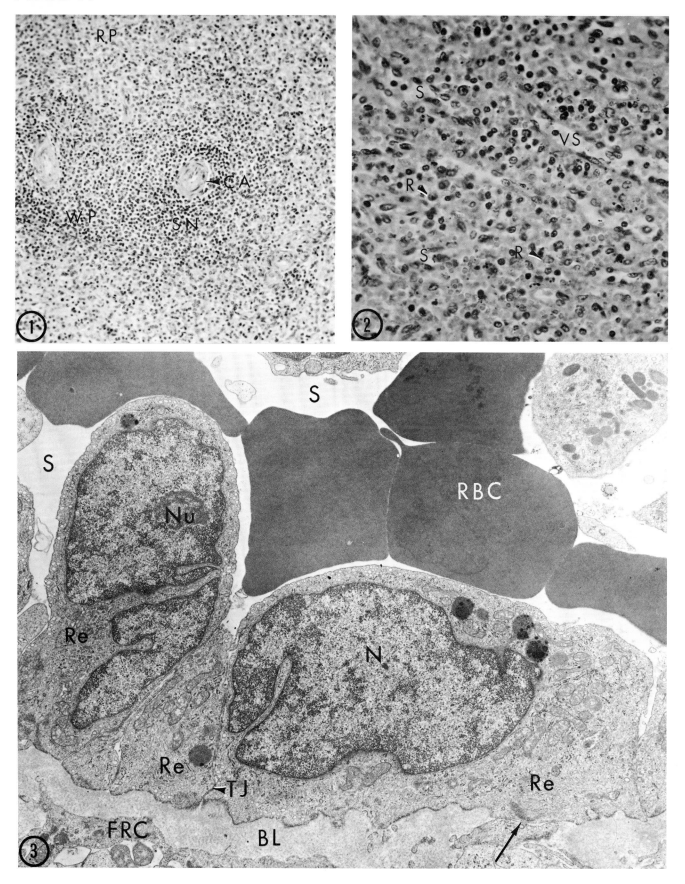

Plate 72 — THYMUS

Figure 1. Photomicrograph of a lobule of thymus. The thymus is a special lymphoid organ derived from the entoderm of the third and fourth pharyngeal pouch. It consists of two lobes surrounded by a capsule (Ca) which extends trabeculae (Tr) into the subjacent cortex. The thymus consists of a dense basophilic cortex surrounding a less dense medulla. The cortex consists of packed thymocytes or lymphocytes that are not clustered into round nodules, as seen in lymph nodules. Since the trabeculae do not extend completely into the medulla, the lobules are not completely separated. The medulla contains numerous small blood vessels and epithelial cells which associate into round clusters called Hassall's corpuscles. (×60)

Figure 2. Photomicrograph of Hassall's corpuscle. A cluster of epithelial cells (EC), surrounded by a basal lamina (BL), is included within a field of lymphocytes (Ly). The central epithelial cells of the corpuscle are partially keratinized, reminiscent of the surface appearance of stratified squamous epithelium. (×600)

Figure 3. Electron micrograph of thymus cortex. Lymphocytes (Ly) in various stages of maturation and larger lymphoblasts (LB) on close inspection are seen to be surrounded by processes of epithelial cells (SE). These epithelial cells replace the reticular cells of other lymph organs; they are not phagocytic nor do they produce a fibrous reticulum. The epithelial cells have lighter-staining nuclei (N) and large nucleoli. Their chromatin is widely dispersed, in contrast to the clumped chromatin seen in the lymphocytes. The cytoplasm contains smooth-surfaced vesicles (V), mitochondria (M), and dense clusters of tonofibrils (TF). By this arrangement of epithelial cells and lymphoid elements, the lymphocytes are generated in spaces separated from the general tissues and tissue fluids by the investing epithelial cells. This protection of forming lymphocytes is unique to the thymus, and may function to protect these cells from influence by exogenous antigens during their development. The epithelial cells are continuous with the epithelial cells of Hassall's corpuscles and are also in contact with the epithelial cells lining the medullary capillaries and capsule and trabecular walls. (×13,000)

PLATE 72

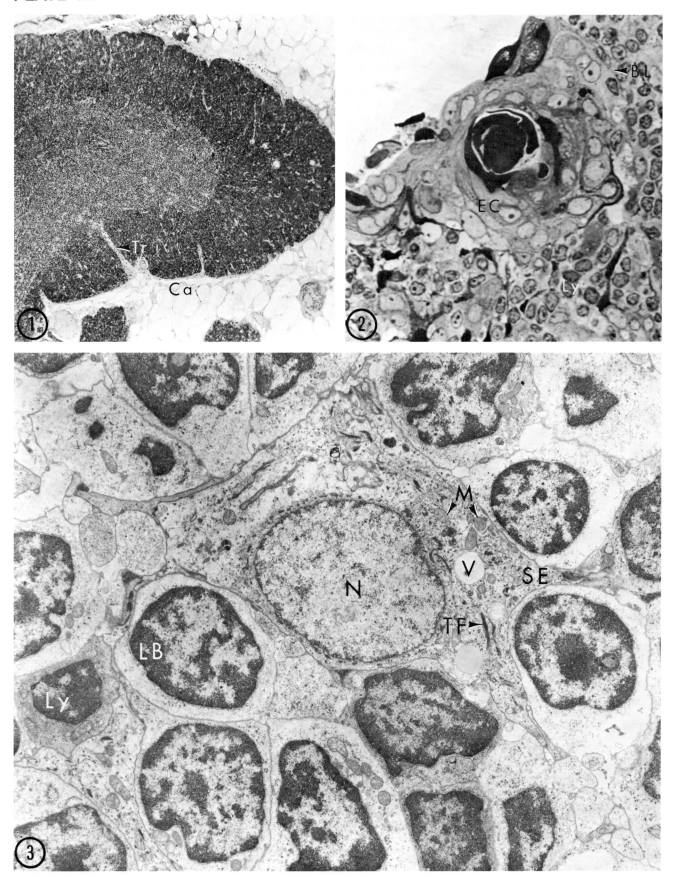

Plate 73 — THYMUS

Figure 1. Electron micrograph of medulla of thymus. Lymphocytes (Ly) produced in the thymus gain access to the circulation by diapedesis through vessel walls. Several structures serve to separate the developing cells from macromolecules in the general circulation. New cells must pass between a row of epithelial cells (EC) surrounding all vessels, through a perivascular space, and between the endothelial cells (EN). In this view, lymphocytes (Ly) are separated from the vessel lumen (L) by thin epithelial cells. Both epithelial and endothelial cells show active pinocytotic activity. ($\times 11,000$)

Figure 2. Electron micrograph of Hassall's corpuscle. Concentric clusters of epithelial cells in the medulla are the Hassall's corpuscles. In this view, the center of the corpuscle (CC) consists of disintegrating keratinized cells. The more peripheral cells contain irregular nuclei (N) and are filled with dense bundles of tonofibrils. Mitochondria (M) and small granules are dispersed between the tonofibrils. Keratohyalin granules do not appear as dense granules, as they do in the skin, but are probably present in the form of the smaller, less dense granules seen in these cells in greater number as the keratinized cells are approached. These keratinized structures may give some support to the medulla, as these cells are continuous with the epithelial cells in the medulla and cortex. ($\times 9,000$)

PLATE 73

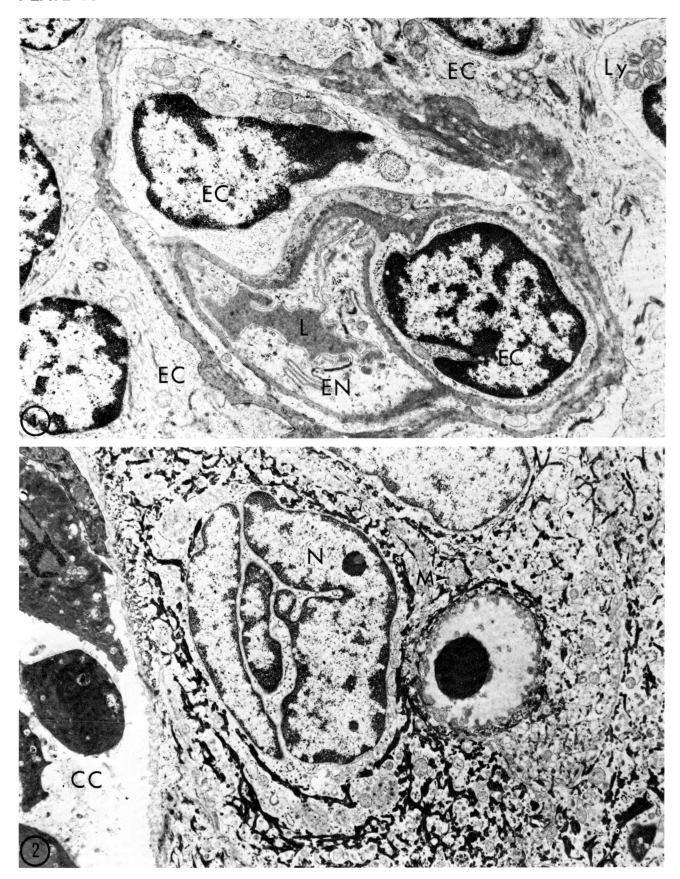

Plate 74 — PALATINE TONSIL

Figure 1. Photomicrograph of palatine tonsil. Tonsils consist of lymph nodules (LN) which may contain germinal centers (GC). The tonsils are covered on one side by mucous membrane which is stratified squamous in the palatine and lingual tonsils. The epithelium invaginates into the underlying lymphoid tissue forming the tonsillar crypts (TC). Deep to the lymph nodules of the tonsil, collagen fibers are condensed but do not form a complete capsule. Afferent lymph vessels are not present. Several lymphocytes move from the nodules and occupy the subepithelial connective tissue. (×70)

Figure 2. Photomicrograph of epon-embedded palatine tonsil. The stratified squamous epithelium (SSE) rests upon a basal lamina (BL). The characteristic layers of this epithelium are present although the stratum granulosum is not prominent. The outer surface is sparsely keratinized. A lymphocyte is seen in the intercellular spaces of the epithelium. Capillaries and general connective-tissue cells along with some lymphocytes occupy the lamina propria (LP). Nuclei of maturing lymphocytes are smaller and darker than the reticulocytes (Re) of the nodule. (×375)

Figure 3. Electron micrograph of palatine tonsil. Squamous epithelial cells of the stratum germinativum rest upon a thin basal lamina (BL). Adjacent cells are separated by a wide intercellular space (IS) into which several epithelial cell processes are extended. Few desmosomes are seen. The cytoplasm of a leukocyte (Le) is seen in this intercellular space on the epithelial side of the basal lamina. Other leukocytes are found in the subjacent collagenous lamina propria (LP). Fibroblasts (F), capillaries (C), and a venule (Ve) are present. The connective-tissue fibers are loosely woven and randomly oriented, facilitating exit of the lymphocytes from the nodule. (×8,000)

162

PLATE 74

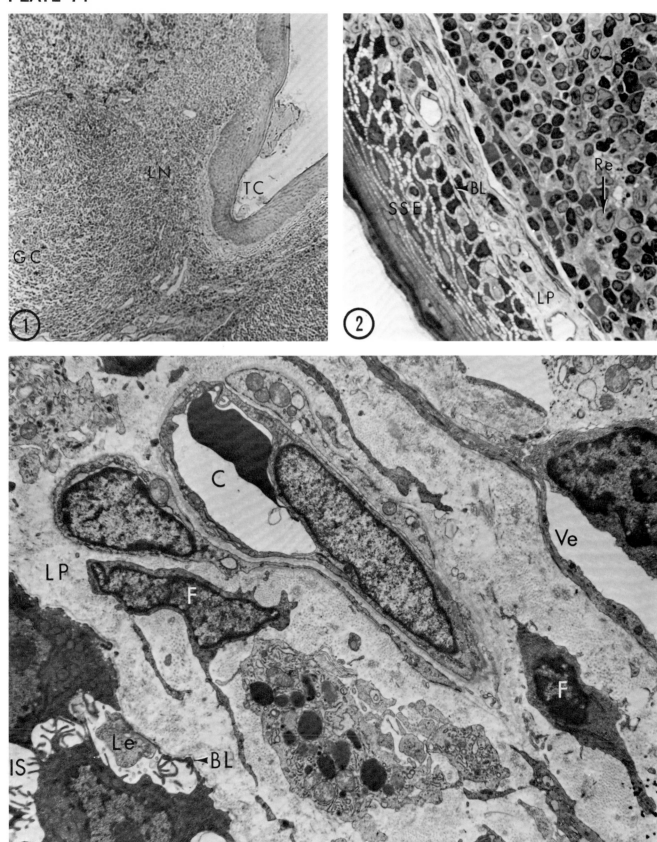

PLATE 81

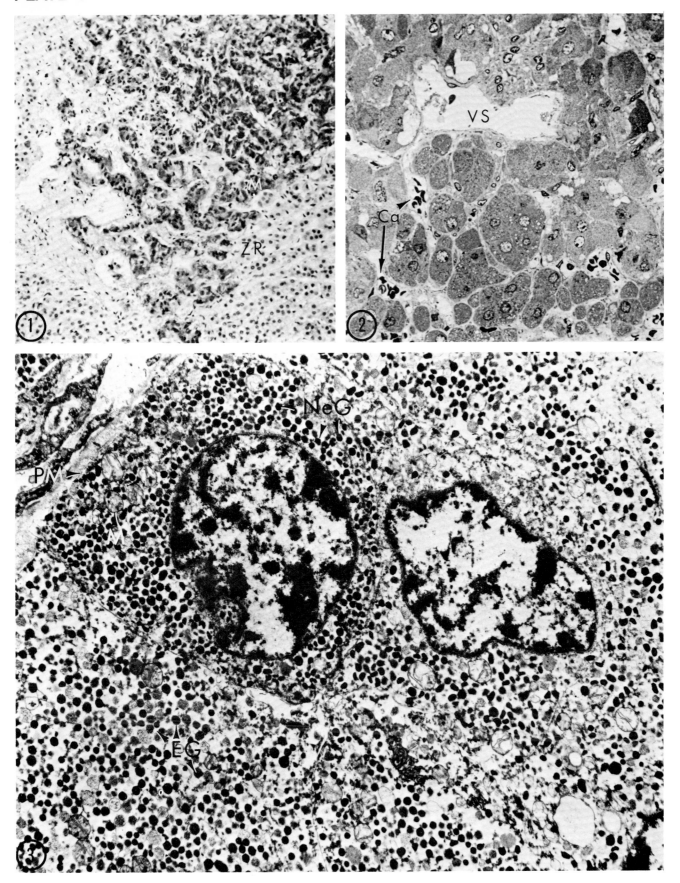

Plate 82 — TESTIS: LEYDIG CELL

Figure 1. Photomicrograph of H&E-stained seminiferous tubule of testis. The seminiferous tubules (ST) contain an irregular lumen (L) and are limited on their outer surface by a basal lamina. The area between adjacent tubules consists of areolar tissue in which many blood vessels (BV) are distributed. Clusters of large rounded cells, the cells of Leydig (Le), are found in this areolar tissue. (×220)

Figure 2. Photomicrograph of plastic thin section of Leydig cells located in the areolar tissue between seminiferous tubules. The nuclei are rounded and some show a prominent dark nucleolus. The cytoplasm contains small basophilic granules. Occasional light spaces are seen which have a crystalline profile. These are the negative images of the crystals of Reinke (R). They appear as elongated prisms containing a crystalline lattice with spacing of about 19 mμ. (×600)

Figure 3. Electron micrograph of interstitial cells of testis. A binucleated cell of Leydig (Le) occupies the center of the field. Sections of adjacent cells of Leydig are also seen, separated from each other by collagen fibrils (Co). The mitochondria of these cells are small and usually round, although some tubular forms are seen. The cytoplasm contains smooth endoplasmic reticulum (SR) which is found throughout the cell. Small irregular dense heterogeneous pigment granules (P) are present. These may contain lipid or a brown pigment, but they are not identical to lipofuscin granules. Small rounded homogeneous granules are present in the cytoplasm and may represent the testosterone moiety. Blood vessels, nerves (N) and fibroblasts (F) are also found in this interstitial region. (×8,400)

180

PLATE 82

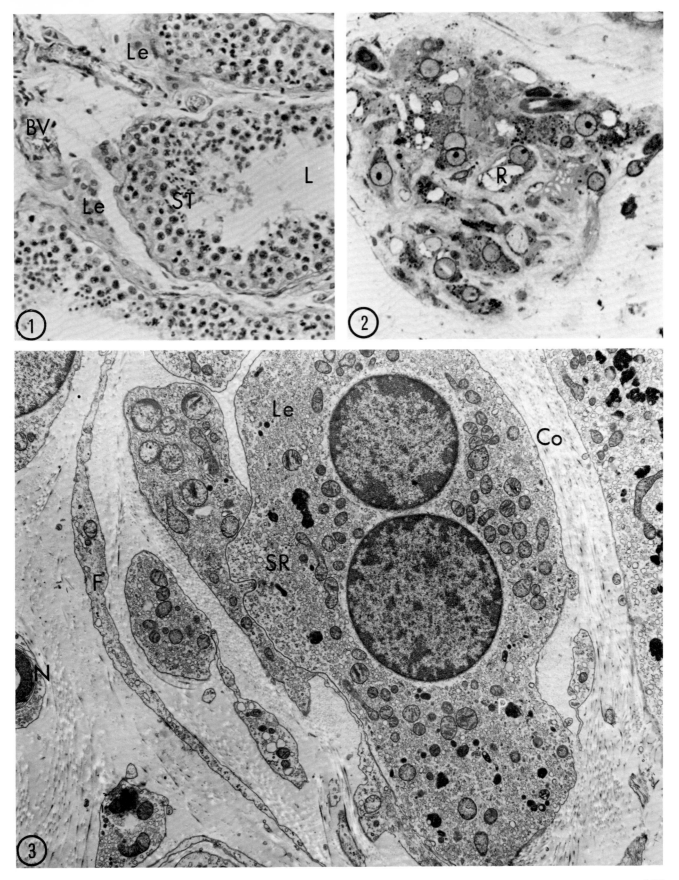

Plate 83 – CORPUS LUTEUM

Figure 1.   Photomicrograph of corpus luteum. Following ovulation, the residual follicular cells and the theca interna collapse into the void left by the ovum and corona radiata. The follicular cells enlarge, become rounded, and fill with lipoid. They are called follicular or granulosa-lutein (FL) cells. The smaller cells of the theca interna also accumulate lipoid droplets and are called theca-lutein cells (TL). Numerous capillaries invade both the theca and granulosa-lutein areas, separating them into clumps and cords. ($\times$150)

Figure 2.   Photomicrograph of epon-embedded corpus luteum. The follicular lutein cells (FL) are large, rounded, and contain an abundance of lipoid. Capillaries (Ca) course between the lutein cells which are also separated by residual fibrin formed following ovulation. The theca-lutein cells (TL) are surrounded by a more fibrous stroma and are smaller than the follicular lutein cells. The outer fibrous theca externa retains its shape and its cells contain lesser amounts of lipoid. ($\times$375)

Figure 3.   Electron micrograph of follicular lutein cells. The follicular cells remaining in the ovary after ovulation become larger and polyhedral; they are arranged in clumps and cords separated by capillaries, fibrin and some collagen fibrils. The nucleus is condensed and contains a large nucleolus (Nu). The cytoplasm is filled with lipoid bodies the contents of which are washed out in routine tissue processing. Other granules are present which are not washed out. These persisting granules are believed to be lipochromes (Lc) consisting of carotenoids. Lipochrome granules autofluoresce and are probably responsible for the yellow color of the corpus luteum in fresh tissue. Negative images of crystalline inclusions (CI) are also present in the cytoplasm. The mitochondria are spherical and contain many tubular cristae arranged in a manner similar to the cristae in cells of the adrenal cortex. Free ribosomes, small Golgi complexes, and both smooth- and rough-surfaced endoplasmic reticulum are present.

   Theca-lutein cells degenerate following each menstrual cycle. Degeneration is accompanied by fatty infiltration, pyknosis of the nucleus, and an increase in acid phosphatases. Connective-tissue cells proliferate and secrete collagen as the lutein cells degenerate, ultimately producing a small corpus albicans. ($\times$7,200)

Figure 4.   Electron micrograph of theca-lutein cells. These cells (TLC) develop from stromal cells (SC). Theca-lutein cells are smaller than granulosa or follicular lutein cells and have a more irregular profile. Cytoplasmic processes often extend from these cells into the surrounding collagenous connective tissue (CT). Lipoid inclusions (L), lipochrome granules (Lc), and negative images of crystals (CI) are also prominent in theca-lutein cells. Small Golgi complexes, spherical mitochondria, smooth-surfaced endoplasmic reticulum and free ribosomes occupy the scanty cytoplasm between lipoid bodies. The mitochondrial cristae of theca-lutein cells also show a tubular arrangement. These cells show degenerative changes during the menstrual cycle in the absence of pregnancy. Degeneration of both follicular and theca-lutein cells is accompanied by degeneration of the outer thecal layer, forming a glassy membrane around the forming corpus albicans. ($\times$7,200)

182

PLATE 83

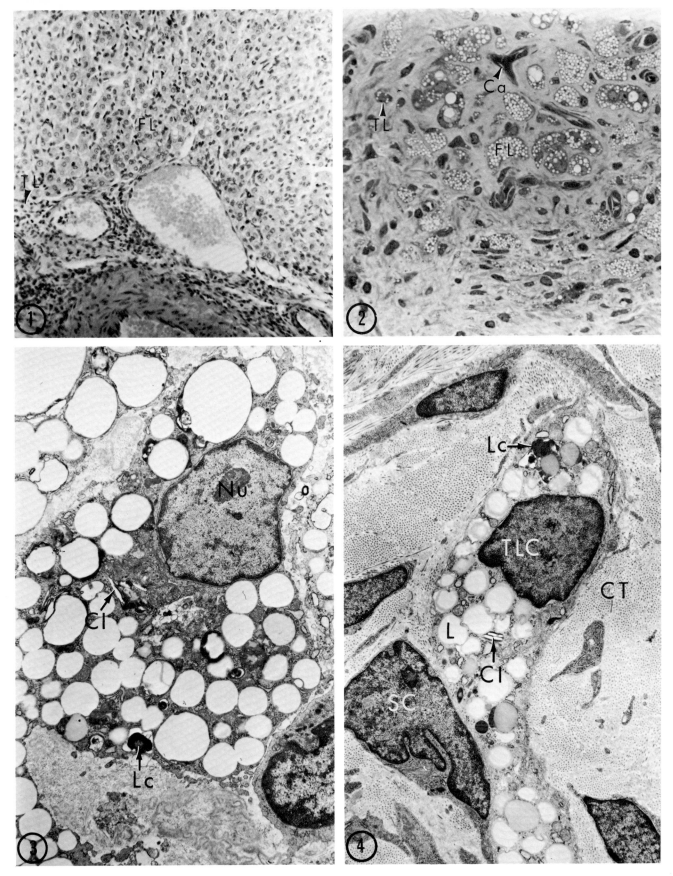

Plate 84 — ISLETS OF LANGERHANS: A CELLS AND B CELLS

Figure 1. Electron micrograph of pancreatic islets of Langerhans. The islets are separated from the exocrine portion of the pancreas by a thin basal lamina. Numerous blood vessels are found both around and within the islets and serve as routes of secretion transport, as no ducts are found within the islets. Two principle cell types are found in the islets: the alpha (A) and beta (B) cells. Other cell types have been identified by special staining but probably represent precursors of the A and B cells.

The A cells (A) are small and have a nucleus (N) which is smaller and more granular than that of the B cells. The cytoplasm of the A cells is filled with dense round granules surrounded by a finely granular cytoplasm. These granules have an outer limiting membrane which is not separated from the contained electron-dense component. The granules are alcohol soluble. Occasional large empty vesicles (V) are found. A few membranes of rough endoplasmic reticulum are scattered in the cytoplasm. A Golgi complex (G) is present, as are numerous small elongated or club-shaped mitochondria (M). The plasma membranes of adjacent cells are close but are not joined by desmosomes or tight junctions.

The beta cells (B) are larger than the alpha cells and their cytoplasm does not have the finely granular osmophilic nature of the alpha cells. Mitochondria are not prominent. Membranes of rough endoplasmic reticulum (ER) are sparse and widely scattered. Large clear vesicles (V) are also found in these cells. The specific granules of beta cells contain insulin. These granules are limited by a membrane which is usually separated from the osmophilic contents. The osmophilic material often has a crystalline configuration (see insert). (×10,600 and ×19,300)

PLATE 84

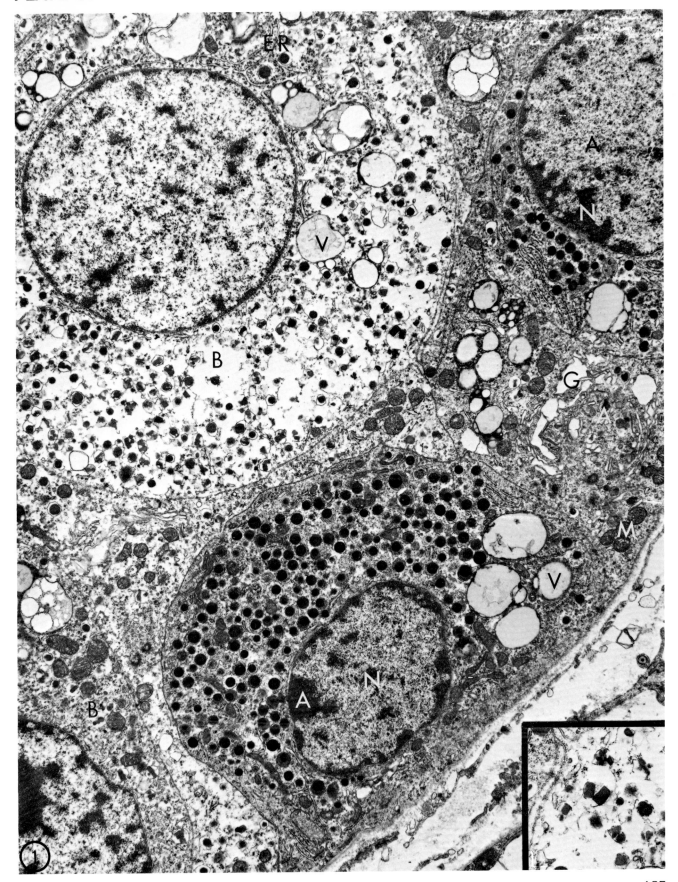

Male Reproductive System

Plate 85 — SPERMATOGENESIS

Figure 1. Photomicrograph of periphery of testis. The outer surface of the testis is covered with a fibrous tunica albuginea (TA) overlying the vascular tunica vasculosa (V), a layer of loose connective tissue. A peritoneal diverticulum, the tunica vaginalis, folds over the albuginea but is not seen in this figure. The testis is divided into pyramidal-shaped lobules by connective-tissue septa which are invaginations of the tunica albuginea. The apex of the lobule terminates in the mediastinal region. Each lobule contains several coiled tubules, the seminiferous tubules (ST), seen here in cross section. They are about 200 μ in diameter. Tubules of adjacent lobules may form anastomoses but ultimately empty into the straight tubules (tubuli recti) connecting with the rete testis. ($\times$130)

Figure 2. Photomicrograph of periphery of seminiferous tubules. Spermatogenesis occurs within the walls of the seminiferous tubules, the outer limits of which are bounded by a basal lamina (BL). The primordial cells, the spermatogonia (Sg), are in contact with the basal lamina. Two stages of spermatogonia are recognized. The A cell, which is about 12 μ in diameter, has a finely granular nucleus with an eccentric nucleolus. These divide mitotically to form A and B cells, the B cells having a more granular chromatin pattern and a central nucleolus. The latter cells have more abundant organelles and will divide mitotically to form primary spermatocytes. Interstitial cells of Leydig (L) are found between the tubules. ($\times$600)

Figure 3. Electron micrograph of seminiferous tubule. A type A spermatogonium (Sg) contacts the basal lamina (BL). This cell contains a nucleus with an eccentric nucleolus (Nu). The cytoplasm contains few organelles other than mitochondria (M) and vesicles of smooth-surfaced endoplasmic reticulum (SR). A part of a Sertoli cell (Se) rests upon the basal lamina and surrounds the spermatogonium and the adjacent primary spermatocytes (PS). The latter cells are larger, have larger nuclei and more SR tubules, and may show a small Golgi complex. These cells show varying phases of nuclear chromatin distribution as they prepare for reduction division. Following the joining of chromosome pairs into interwoven tetrads (a process termed synapsis) chromosome pairs are separated at the division plane with half the intact chromosomes going to each cell, producing the haploid number of chromosomes. The resultant smaller cells are the secondary spermatocytes, shown on Plate 86. ($\times$8,200)

PLATE 85

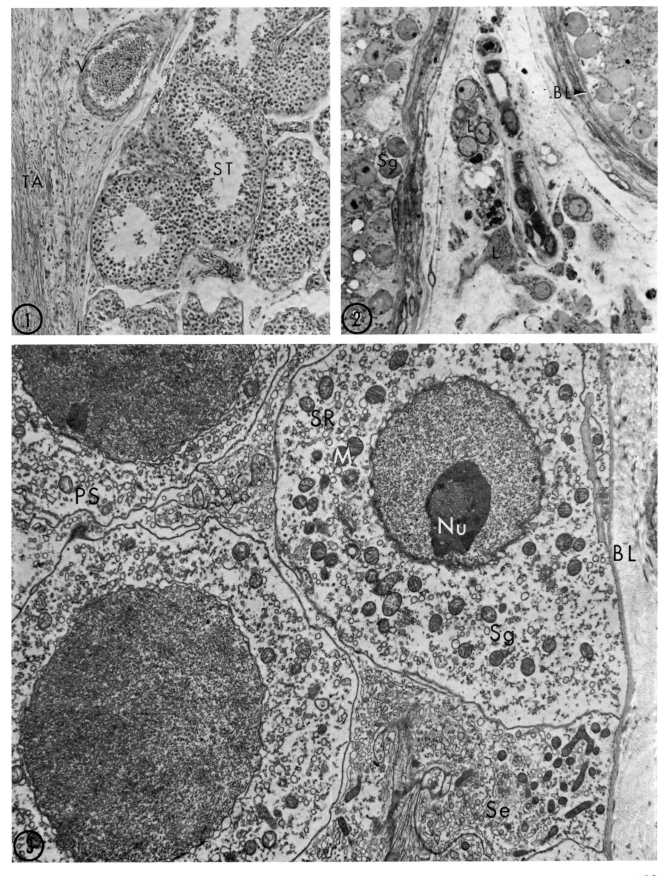

Plate 86 — TESTIS: SERTOLI CELLS

Figure 1. Photomicrograph of plastic section of seminiferous tubule. The outer limit of the tubule consists of a basal lamina surrounded by collagen. Fibroblasts (F) are found in the surrounding collagen. The large clear cells resting upon the inner surface of the basal lamina are the spermatogonia (Sg). Successive stages of spermatogenesis, the spermatocytes (Sc), are represented by the rounded cells situated in the midwall of the tubule. These cells are surrounded by cells with numerous thin cytoplasmic extensions, the Sertoli cells (Se). The mitochondria of the Sertoli cells are small, numerous, and stain deeply with paragon stain. The cells that proximate the lumen (L) are in various stages of spermiogenesis. ($\times$600)

Figure 2. Electron micrograph of Sertoli cell. The cytoplasm of the Sertoli cells contains three definitive features. The mitochondria (M) are small and tubular shaped. The cytoplasm is filled with membranes of smooth endoplasmic reticulum (SR). Special membranous structures consisting of concentrically arranged membranes, the annulate lamellae (AL), are abundant. These lamellae resemble a coiled nuclear membrane with repeating annuli, the equivalent of nuclear pores. The annulate lamellae appear to bud off to form smooth endoplasmic reticulum. An annulus is indicated at the arrow. ($\times$12,140)

Figure 3. Electron micrograph of Sertoli cell. The nucleus (N) of this cell has a typical cleft. Two nucleoli are present. The chromatin pattern is finely granular and does not show prominent clumps. The shape of the cell is irregular. One part of a cytoplasmic process can be traced to the basal lamina (BL). This process and a second one completely circle a spermatogonium (Sg). Cytoplasmic processes of these cells surround every cell undergoing differentiation into spermatozoa and thus must at least partially regulate the progression of cells toward the lumen. The cytoplasm contains abundant vesicles of smooth endoplasmic reticulum (SR). Irregular-shaped lipid bodies (L) are present, as are other membrane vesicles of unknown content. Some pigment granules (P) are scattered in the cytoplasm. The mitochondria (M) are smaller and more elongated than those of the spermatogonia. ($\times$8,500)

PLATE 86

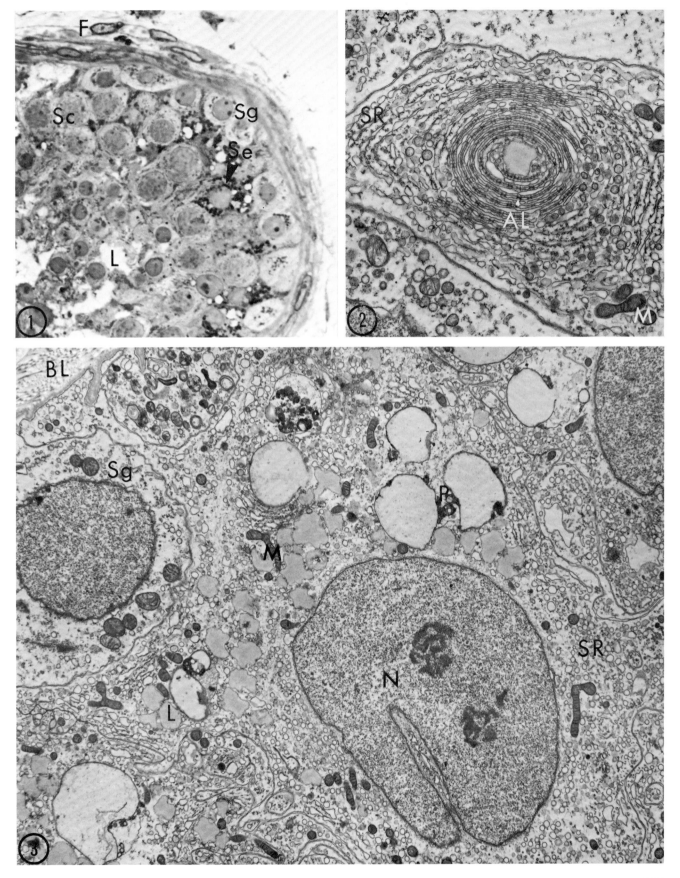

Plate 87 – SPERMIOGENESIS

Figure 1. Electron micrograph of secondary spermatocytes. The secondary spermatocytes (SS) result from the reduction division of the larger primary spermatocytes. The secondary spermatocytes are small round cells with condensed nuclei (N). They quickly divide by mitosis (maturation division) to form spermatids. These latter cells do not divide further but undergo a metamorphosis into spermatozoa, a process called spermiogenesis. The secondary spermatocytes have an abundance of smooth-surfaced endoplasmic reticulum and develop a prominent Golgi complex (G). The spermatocytes are surrounded by thin processes of Sertoli cells (SC), the mitochondria of which are smaller and more dense than those of the spermatocytes. ($\times$4,600)

Figure 2. Electron micrograph of early spermatids. Spermatids are about 9 μ in diameter and have a spherical nucleus (N) and a prominent Golgi complex (G). An electron-dense material accumulates within vesicles of the Golgi complex and a material of comparable density begins to accumulate on the edge of the nuclear membrane on one side. The dense granule which forms here is the acrosomal granule (A). This granule increases in size, is PAS positive, and obtains additional material from vesicles of the Golgi complex. Two parts of an acrosome are distinguished: the amorphous electron-dense acrosome and an outer limiting membrane, the head cap (HC), which fuses with the nuclear membrane at the nuclear equator. ($\times$6,600)

Figure 3. Electron micrograph of maturing spermatid. In this figure, the head cap (HC) extends from the acrosomal granule (A) to the nuclear equator. The Golgi complex is reduced in size. A few mitochondria (M) and smooth endoplasmic reticulum (SER) are present. Centrioles will attach to the nuclear membrane at the arrows. ($\times$9,000)

Figure 4. Electron micrograph of a mature spermatozoon. The nucleus, head cap and acrosome form the head (H); the centriole, flagellum, peripheral fibers, mitochondria (M) and membrane form the midbody; and the axial filaments (AF) (flagellum), seven peripheral fibers, and outer membrane continue as the tail of the spermatozoon. The mature human sperm thus consists of a "head" and "midbody" about 4 μ long to which a 30 to 50 μ "tail" is attached. Sperm attain motility upon maturation in the epididymus and can move at rates of 50 μ per second. ($\times$7,800)

192

PLATE 87

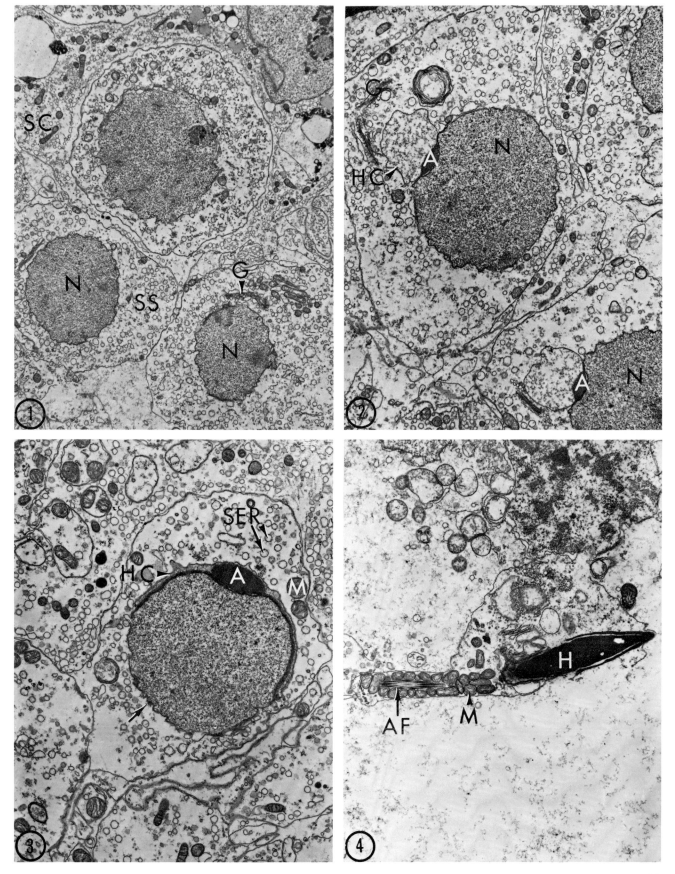

Plate 88 – DUCTUS EPIDIDYMIS

Figure 1.   Photomicrograph of tubules of epididymis. The ductuli efferentes empty into the epididymis, which is outside of the tunica albuginea. The epididymis has head and body segments, and terminates in a tail emptying into the ductus deferens. The epididymis consists of well-oriented epithelial cells, with each columnar cell evenly matching the length of its neighbor. The tubules are surrounded by a fibrous stroma (S) and circularly arranged smooth muscle fibers. The lumen (L) is thus smooth and regular. Extensions of nonmotile cytoplasmic processes, the stereocilia, project into the lumen. A group of pyramidal-shaped epithelial cells is interposed between the tall columnar cells, so the epithelium is pseudostratified columnar. (×200)

Figure 2.   Photomicrograph of plastic section of epididymis. Connective tissue and blood vessels are seen below the basement membrane (B). Two rows of epithelial nuclei are seen. The deep nuclei are dark and rounded, and contain a small nucleolus. The nuclei (N) of the columnar shaped cells are irregular, show extensive folding, and contain several dense nucleoli. The lumen has stereocilia around which rounded cytoplasmic residual bodies and spermatozoa are seen. The outer wall has some circularly arranged smooth muscle increasing in thickness at the vas deferens, where the muscle becomes the most prominent feature of the ductule. (×600)

Figure 3.   Electron micrograph of lumen portion of epithelial cells of epididymis. Stereocilia (Sc) are elongate structures with thick bases. Tight junctions (TJ) unite cell membranes at the lumen. Secretory vesicles (V), a prominent Golgi complex (G), and small granular mitochondria are present. (×5,300)

Figure 4.   Electron micrograph of basilar portion of cells seen in Figure 3. In this figure, the basement membrane (B) is at the top of the field. The nucleus and cytoplasm of a basal cell (BC) are seen at the basement membrane. The columnar cell is below this and contains a complexly folded nucleus (N). The nuclei contain prominent nucleoli. (×5,200)

194

PLATE 88

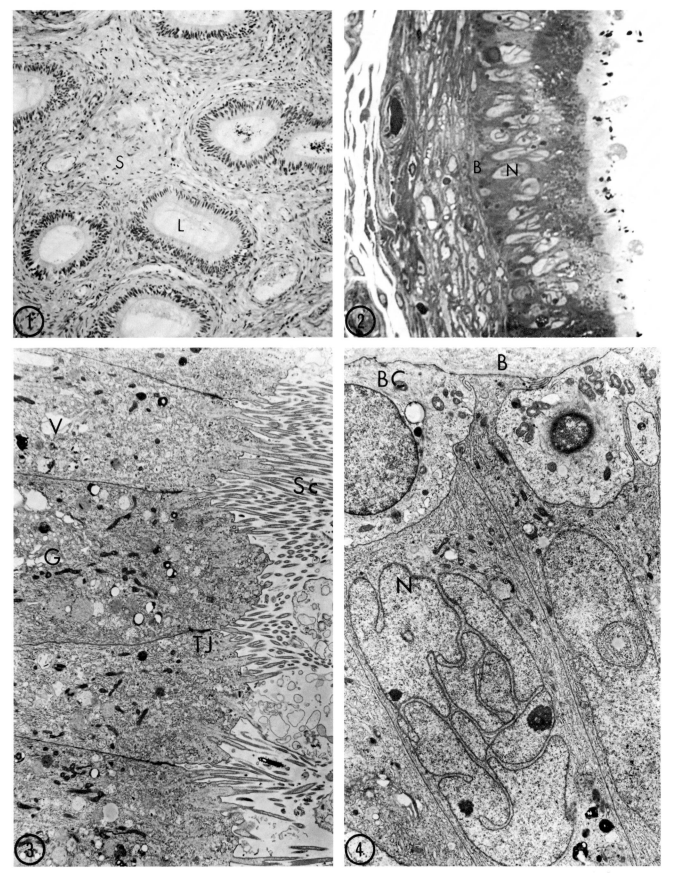

Plate 89 — DUCTULI EFFERENTES

Figure 1. The ductuli efferentes are 10 to 15 ductules connecting the thin-walled rete testis with the epididymis outside the testis. In this photomicrograph, portions of two tubules are seen. The epithelial cells lining the tubule lumen (L) are primarily columnar, but some shorter cells are interposed between the columnar cells. The tubular walls contain some smooth muscle, and elastic and collagen fibers. Partial contraction of the circular muscle fibers, and the alternating heights of the epithelial cells, cause the lining to show an irregular luminal surface. ($\times$180)

Figure 2. Photomicrograph of a plastic section of the ductuli efferentes. The lumen (L) is lined with epithelial cells, many of which show a fine microvillus border. The nuclei of these cells have a prominent cleft. The cells rest upon a basal lamina (BL), and their walls consist of smooth muscle fibers, collagen, and some elastic fibers. ($\times$600)

Figure 3. Electron micrograph of epithelial cells of tubule. Cells of differing heights rest upon the basal lamina (BL). A fibroblast (F) is seen immediately below the basal lamina and is surrounded by collagen fibrils. The luminal surface (L) of the columnar-shaped cells shows two features. The cells have numerous small microvilli (Mv). Some cells have a single motile cilium (Ci). The nuclei (N) have a prominent cleft. The mitochondria (M) are small and tubular and are found throughout the cytoplasm. A Golgi complex (G) is on the luminal side of the nucleus and is associated with several membrane-bound secretion granules (S). Pigment granules (P) may be present. The rounded epithelial cells (E) rest upon the basal lamina, contain a rounded nucleus (N) and have few organelles. ($\times$6,800)

PLATE 89

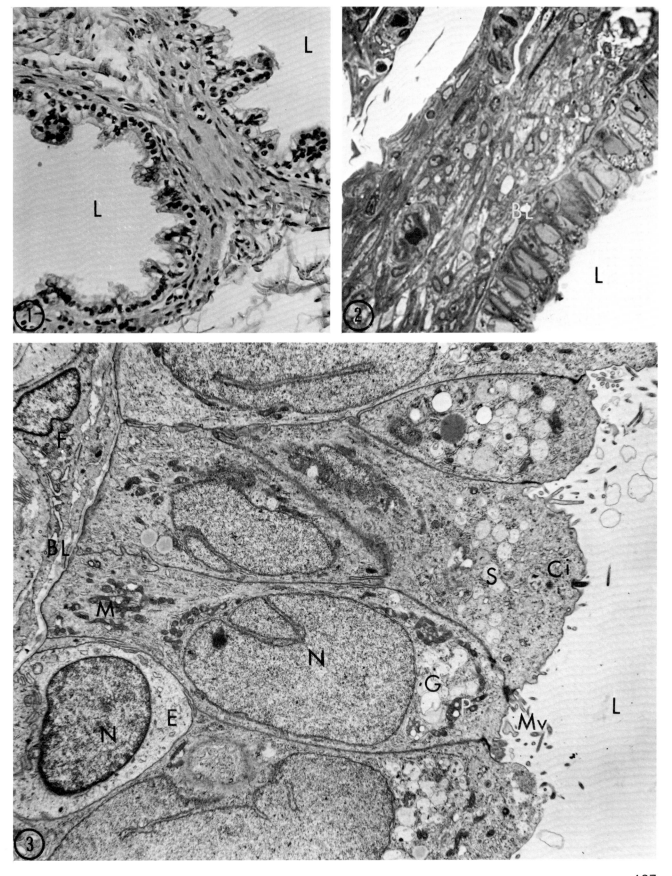

Plate 90 — PROSTATE

Figure 1. Photomicrograph of prostate. Glands of the prostate empty into the V-shaped lumen of the prostatic urethra. The glands are of three different sizes and are arranged around the urethra so that the smallest glands are in the mucosal layer, the next largest occupy the submucosal layer (SM), and the largest prostate glands (PG) are peripherally disposed in the stroma (S). The glands are sacculated and are lined with simple columnar epithelium. The stroma consists of fibrous elements and smooth muscle fibers. (×150)

Figure 2. Photomicrograph of epon-embedded prostate. Glandular units are lined with simple columnar epithelium. More than one layer of cells appear because of the tangential section. The apical part of the cells is filled with secretion vesicles. Three concretions (Co) occupy the lumen of the gland. The stroma consists of collagen fibers and fibroblasts (F). Smooth muscle fibers (MF) course through the fibrous stroma. (×375)

Figure 3. Electron micrograph of prostate epithelium. The epithelial cells rest upon a basal lamina (BL). Collagen fibers (Co) and fibroblasts (F) surround the gland. The epithelial cells are columnar and show both basal and centrally positioned nuclei (N). Small microvilli project from the apical surface. Empty membrane-lined secretion vesicles occupy the apical cytoplasm and are separated by mitochondria and a few membranes of rough-surfaced endoplasmic reticulum. Free ribosomes are abundant in the cytoplasm. A few small dense crystalloids (Cr) are present. The Golgi complex is obscured by the large secretion vesicles. (×9,400)

PLATE 90

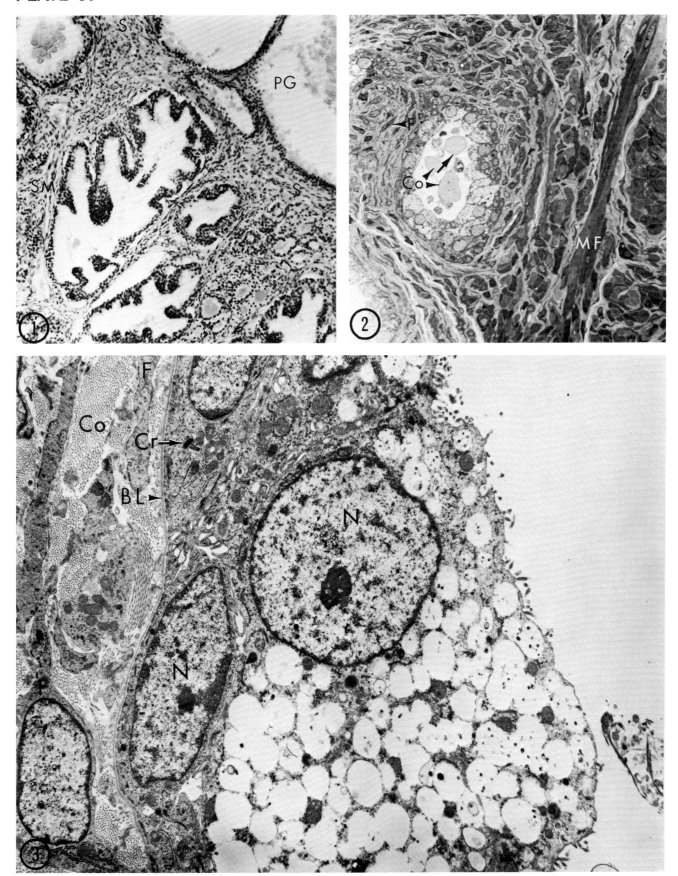

Plate 91 — PROSTATE

Figure 1. Electron micrograph of prostate. The epithelial cells of the prostatic glands are simple cuboidal or simple columnar. The nucleus (N) is oval and is surrounded by cytoplasm filled with secretion vesicles (SV) the contents of which are washed out in routine preparative procedures. These vesicles normally contain high concentrations of acid phosphatase, citric acid, and proteolytic enzymes. Small microvilli protrude into the lumen, which is also occupied by a spherical body or concretion (Co). ($\times 7,700$)

Figure 2. Electron micrograph of prostate concretion. Concretions are described as solid aggregates of prostate secretions which occasionally calcify. They are common in the prostates of older men. The concretion consists of lamellae of a fibrillar mat in which the fibrils vary in density and direction in adjacent layers. Arrows indicate a lamellar boundary. A ground substance binds the fibrils into a dense mat. Numerous membranous vesicles are trapped within the fibrils. This concretion is very similar to the perichondrocyte capsule seen in the lacunar walls of elastic cartilage. ($\times 25,000$)

PLATE 91

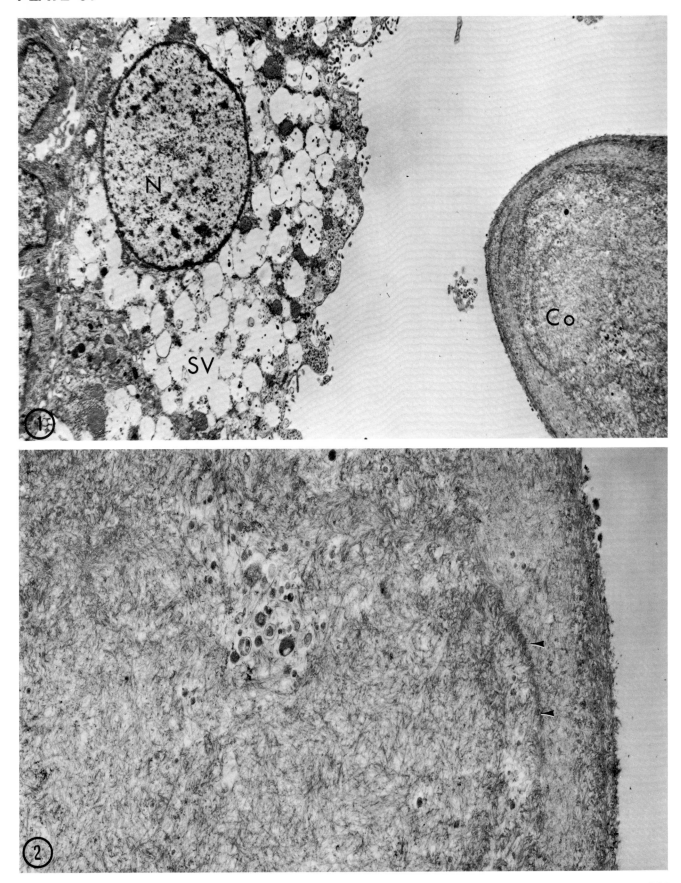

Female Reproductive System

Plate 92 — OVARY: PRIMARY FOLLICLE

Figure 1. Photomicrograph of ovary cortex. The ovary consists of a cortex and a medulla. The surface of the ovary is covered with a layer of simple cuboidal epithelium called the germinal epithelium (GE) although it apparently does not function to produce oogonia. The connective tissue is called the ovarian stroma (S) and consists of large numbers of cells arranged randomly. The stroma just inside the germinal epithelium is less cellular and forms the tunica albuginea (TA). The medulla consists of areolar tissue and several convoluted arteries and veins. Several primary follicles (PF) lie in the stroma and consist of a primary oocyte and surrounding follicular or granulosa cells. (×150)

Figure 2. Photomicrograph of epon-embedded ovarian cortex. Primary follicles (PF) are surrounded by a cellular stroma (S). The follicles are composed of a primary oocyte and thin follicular cells. With further development, the oocytes enlarge and the flattened follicular cells increase in number and assume a cuboidal to columnar shape. The primary oocytes complete their first meiotic division when development of the follicle is sufficient for them to rupture from the ovarian surface during ovulation. (×375)

Figure 3. Electron micrograph of primary follicle. The primary oocyte is relatively large (35 to 50 μ) and contains a large electron-lucent nucleus (N). The nucleus contains widely dispersed chromatin and a prominent nucleolus which changes with development. The nuclear membrane has several prominent nuclear pores. Mitochondria (M) occupy a juxtanuclear position. Smooth-surfaced endoplasmic reticulum (SER) is scattered in the cytoplasm as are small dense yolk granules. The follicular cells are squamous shaped and are closely adherent to the oocyte plasma membrane. A thin basal lamina (BL) separates the primary follicle from the surrounding cellular stroma (S). (×6,000)

204

PLATE 98

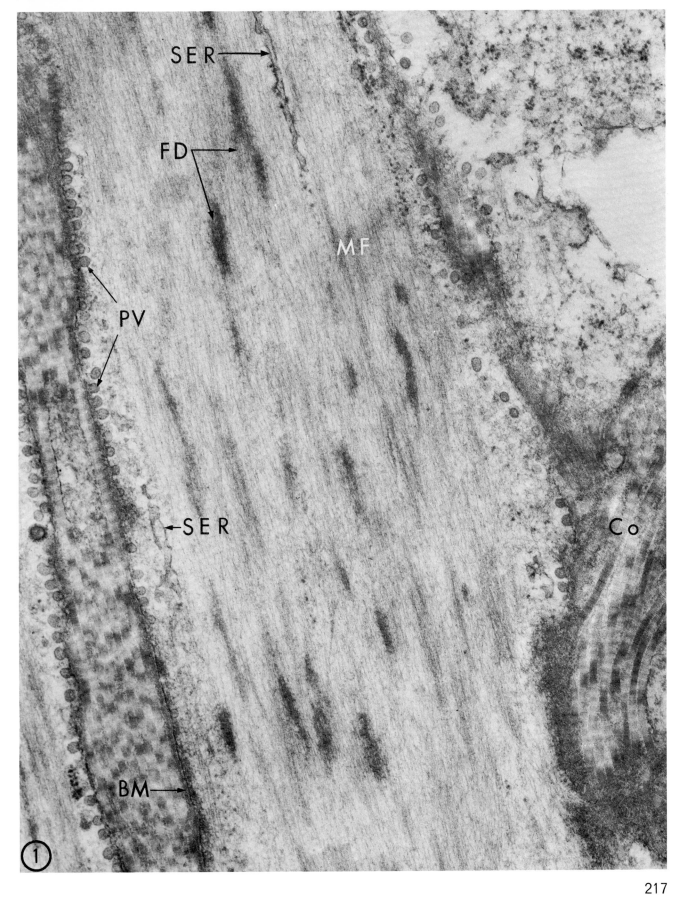

Plate 99 — MAMMARY GLAND

Figure 1. Photomicrograph of resting mammary gland. Glands emptying into one of the lactiferous ducts of the nipple comprise a lobe of the breast. Lobes are further divided into lobules separated by fibrous connective tissue (FCT) in which adipose cells are trapped and supported. In the resting mammary gland, the lobules, of ducts and parenchymal cells, are small and widely scattered; they consist of branching intralobular ducts (ID) terminating in small dilations. The epithelium of the ducts consists of two layers of cells containing oval nuclei which may be oriented differently in the two layers. The entire lobule is surrounded by fibrous connective tissue with widely distributed fibroblasts. An interlobular duct (D) is seen at the right of the field. Within the lobule, the connective tissue is cellular and corresponds to the papillary layer of the dermis from which it originated. (×150)

Figure 2. Photomicrograph of epon-embedded lobule of resting mammary gland. Intralobular ducts are surrounded by a thin basal lamina (BL) and are separated by fibrous connective tissue containing numerous fibroblasts (F). The ducts may consist of two layers of cells. The nuclei are oval, contain nucleoli, and are oriented so that the axis of the inner nuclei may parallel the lumen border; however, many have round nuclei and show no spatial orientation. (×375)

Figure 3. Electron micrograph of mammary gland duct. The nucleus contains finely condensed chromatin. A large nucleolus (Nu) is characteristic and may occupy any part of the nucleus. The free margin has microvilli and junctional complexes (JC) are seen between contiguous cells bordering the lumen. The basal surface of the cell is irregular and rests upon a thin basal lamina (BL). These cells contain an abundance of free ribosomes but rough-surfaced endoplasmic reticulum is present. A Golgi complex (GC) and centriole occupy the apical cytoplasm in the cell on the right. The second, outer cell layer is represented here by one cell attached to the surface cells by desmosomes (De). The nucleus of the latter cell is elongate and parallel to the basal lamina, contrary to the orientation ordinarily described. (×11,200)

PLATE 99

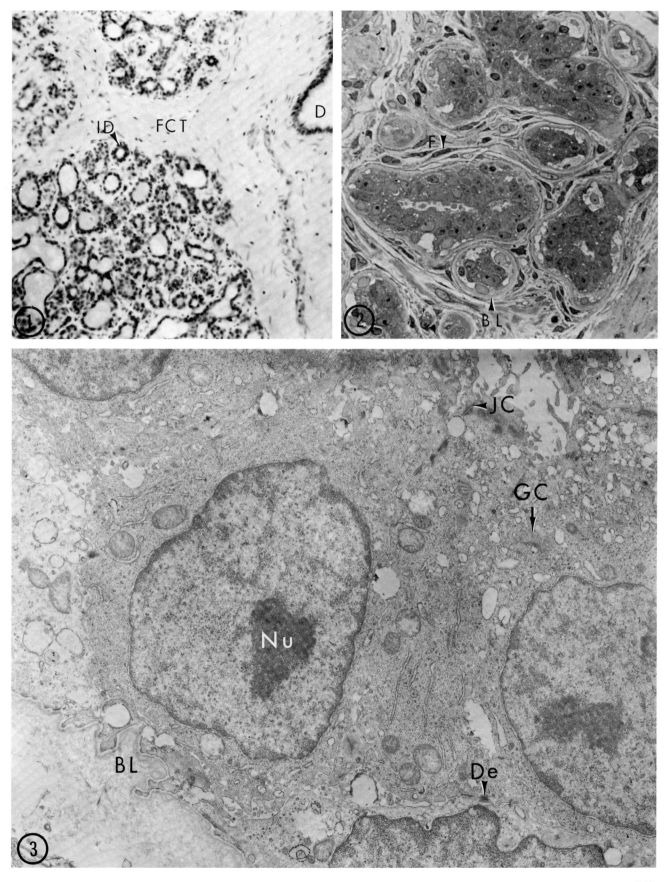

Plate 100 — MAMMARY GLAND

Figure 1.   Electron micrograph of resting mammary gland. This micrograph is from the dilated terminal end of an intralobular duct. Two layers of cells are present but the cells near the lumen are larger and have a columnar shape. The nuclei are centrally positioned. Microvilli (Mv) are abundant on some cells but absent on others. Junctional complexes (JC) unite adjacent cells at their contiguous apical boundaries. A Golgi complex (GC) lies in the apical cytoplasm. Free ribosomes are widely distributed but tubules of rough-surfaced endoplasmic reticulum (ER) are also seen in all parts of the cell. Some of the tubules form cisternae. The apical portions of the cells lining the lumen and the peripheral cytoplasm of the basal cells contain tonofilaments. A basal lamina (BL) occupies the epithelial-connective tissue interface.

Following stimulation by hormones during pregnancy, alveoli lined by columnar cells proliferate, causing the lobules to enlarge and the intralobular ducts to become more widely separated. These secretory cells contain numerous electron-dense secretion granules and lipid bodies. (×12,000)

PLATE 100

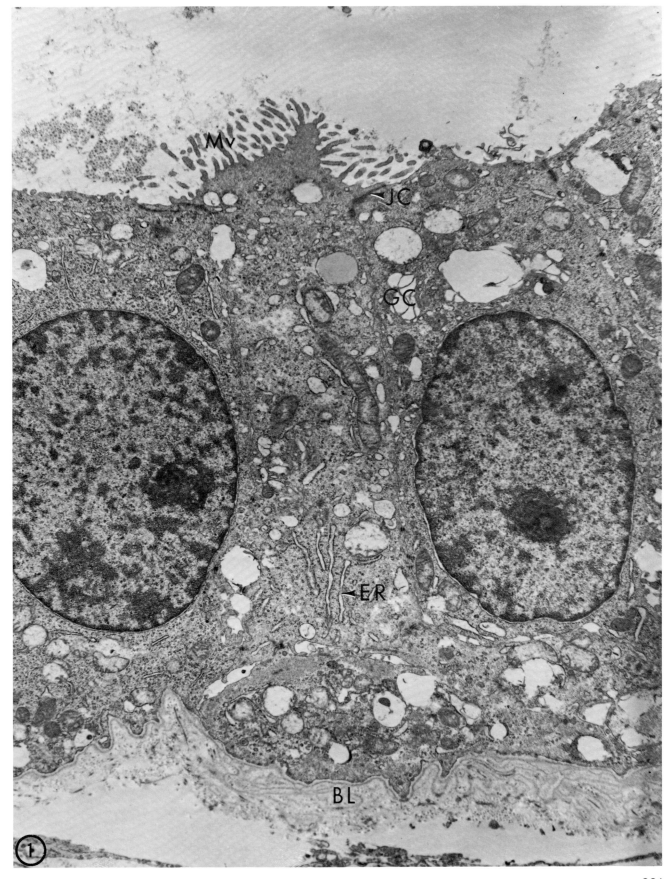

Plate 101 — PLACENTA

Figure 1.   Photomicrograph of placenta. The placenta consists of two components: fetal and maternal. The fetal component consists of a chorionic plate (CP) and branching processes or villi (V) which originate at the chorionic plate and project into spaces through which maternal blood (MB) circulates. Some villi are large and filled with connective-tissue fibers extending back into the decidua basalis, anchoring the chorionic plate to the uterus. Smaller villi are attached by slender connections. ($\times$150)

Figure 2.   Photomicrograph of epon-embedded villus. Blood of the fetal circulation does not communicate directly with maternal blood. Several special cells and structures are interposed between these two circulations. In this figure, a villus (Vi) projects into a maternal blood space (MB). The villi are covered by dark, multinucleated cells, the syncytiotrophoblasts (Sy). These cells also line the maternal blood spaces adjacent to the chorionic plate (CP). A second cell type, which becomes thin and attenuated in the term placenta, is interposed between the syncytiotrophoblast and the mesenchymal tissue in the villus core. This second cell type is the cytotrophoblast (Cy). Capillaries (C) circulating fetal blood are supported by the mesenchymal tissue of the villus core. ($\times$375)

Figure 3.   Electron micrograph of chorionic villus. Maternal blood circulates through spaces (MBS) lined by syncytiotrophoblasts (Sy). These cells have dense granular cytoplasm and extend microvilli (Mv) into the maternal blood space. Several nuclei (N) are present in this field but no definitive intercellular boundaries are distinguished. This essentially produces a syncytium of cells lining all maternal blood spaces. Several vacuoles (V) and granules (G) are present on both basal and apical cytoplasm. Mitochondria (M) are small and have few cristae. The syncytial cells are separated from the cytotrophoblasts (Cy) by a narrow space. The cytotrophoblast has thin cytoplasmic plates resembling squamous epithelial cells. The nucleus (N2) shows little heterochromatin formation and is spindle shaped in lateral profile. These cells are cuboidal in the early months of pregnancy and probably produce the syncytiotrophoblasts. A basal lamina (BL) separates the cytotrophoblast from the subjacent areolar tissue. A fetal capillary (FC) is lined by simple squamous endothelium and surrounded by a thin basal lamina. Regulation of maternal-fetal exchange of nutrients, gases, ions, antibodies, etc., is effected by these basal laminae and cells. ($\times$12,300)

PLATE 101

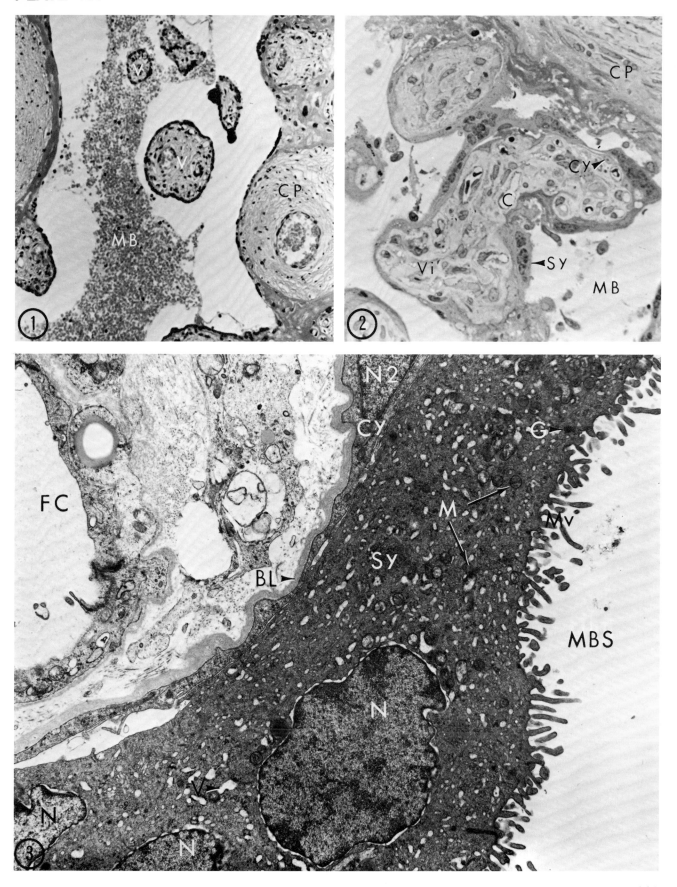

Plate 102 — PLACENTA

Figure 1.   Electron micrograph of term placenta. The fetal circulation is separated from the maternal circulation by endothelial cells, basal lamellae, and two special cell layers: the syncytiotrophoblasts (Sy) and the cytotrophoblasts (Cy). These two cell layers are joined by desmosomes (De). Areas of nonunion of the two cell layers are occupied by microvilli (Mv) of both cell types, although the syncytiotrophoblasts provide most of the microvilli. Microvilli also project from these cells into the maternal blood sinus of the intervillous space. Pinocytotic vesicles (Pv) are seen at the cell margins. The syncytiotrophoblast is a large, flat, multinucleated (N) layer of cells characterized by large vesicles (V) and several small Golgi complexes (G). Mitochondria are large and have few cristae (Cr). Free ribosomes are widely scattered. The cytotrophoblast nucleus is larger and has more finely dispersed chromatin. A nucleolus (Nu) is prominent. These cells do not form a syncytium but are separated individually by plasma membranes (PM). Both free ribosomes and rough-surfaced endoplasmic reticulum (ER) are present. Golgi complexes (G) and mitochondria are small. Microvilli course through the basal lamina (BL) to reach the connective tissues and capillaries of the chorion. ($\times$14,800)

PLATE 102

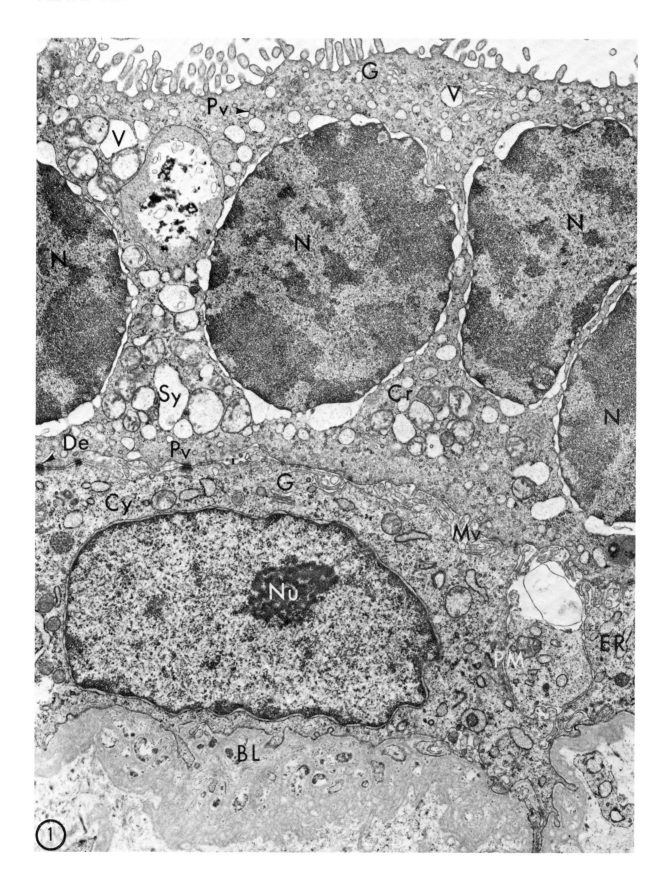

225

Oral Glands

Plate 103 — SALIVARY GLAND

Figure 1.   Photomicrograph of submandibular gland. The salivary glands are compound tubuloalveolar glands. The secretory acini of this submandibular gland consist of either serous cells or mucous cells. The cytoplasm of the serous cells (S) is granular and slightly basophilic. The nuclei of these cells are round and located in the basal cell portion. The mucous cells (M) have a less granular cytoplasm and their nuclei are usually flattened against the basal lamina of the acinus. Occasionally, serous cells cluster at the periphery of the mucous acinus making a demilune (De). An intralobular duct (D) collects saliva from the acini of the lobule. (×150)

Figure 2.   Electron micrograph of secretory acinus of submandibular gland. Secretory cells (S) are separated by intercellular channels into which several cell processes are extended. Interspersed between secretory cells and surrounding the acini at their outer limits are contractile cells called myoepithelial cells (My). These cells have long branching processes and their cytoplasm contains filaments and fusiform densities comparable to those observed in smooth muscle cells. (×8,500)

Figure 3.   Electron micrograph of serous secretory cells. The nucleus (N) has condensed chromatin, contains a prominent nucleolus (Nu), is oval and is situated in that portion of the cell oriented toward the outer limiting basal lamina of the acinus. Rough endoplasmic reticulum (ER) fills the cytoplasm and exhibits a fingerprint type of arrangement. Small mitochondria are scattered between the extensive ER membranes. The secretory granules are membrane limited, generally large, and electron dense. (×8,500)

Figure 4.   Electron micrograph of mucous cells of submandibular gland acinus. The nuclei (N) of these cells are generally close to the cell border. The mucous granules (MG) are made up of a central electron-dense core and a lighter amorphous material which is membrane limited. (×8,600)

228

PLATE 103

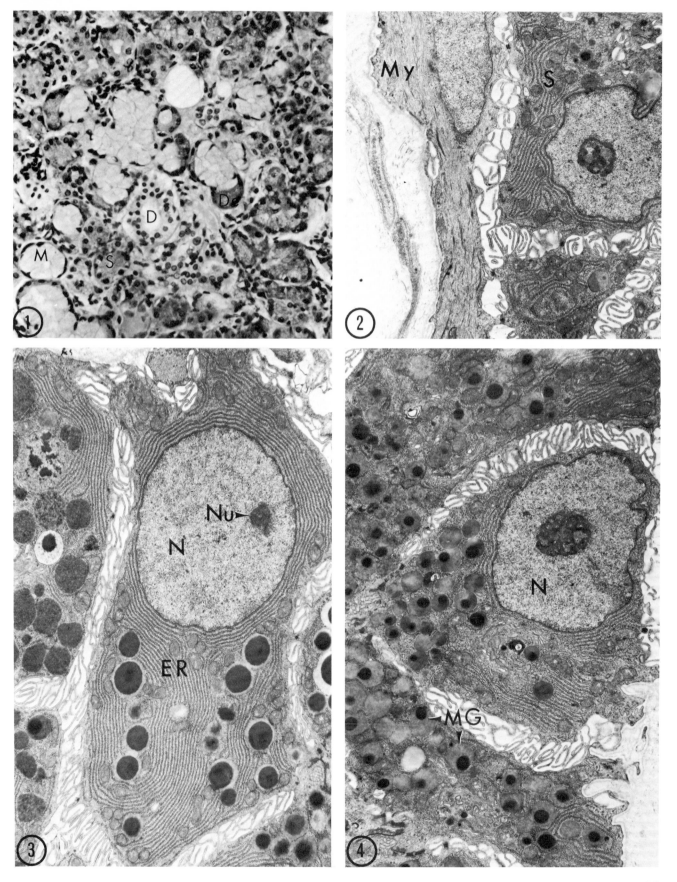

Plate 104 — SALIVARY GLAND DUCTS

Figure 1.   Photomicrograph of lobule of submandibular gland. The secretory acini, both mucous (M) and serous (S), empty into an ordered duct system which begins at the secretory acini as intercalated ducts and then empties into intralobular ducts (I), which in turn ultimately empty into interlobular ducts. ($\times 150$)

Figure 2.   Photomicrograph of epon-embedded section of submandibular gland. Intercalated duct cells (D) continue directly from the cells of the acini (S) in which the secretory granules and the intercellular channels may be resolved. These duct cells show a clear cytoplasm with few organelles. Their nuclei are slightly larger and more centrally placed than those of the acinar cells. ($\times 600$)

Figure 3.   Electron micrograph of duct of submandibular gland. The intercalated ducts are composed of cuboidal cells with oval nuclei (N) and few organelles. Mitochondria and a few membranes of rough endoplasmic reticulum (ER) are included. The cells are closely apposed to their neighbors and junction complexes (J) are seen at the lumen (L) interface. Intercalated ducts empty into striated or secretory ducts. Cells of these ducts appear striated, as their abundant mitochondria (M) are concentrated in rows in the basal portion of these cells. More extensive membranes of rough-surfaced endoplasmic reticulum (ER) are present, indicating a synthetic activity. Parts of two of these cells are included in the top of this figure; thus, this section was made at the duct site where the intercalated duct becomes a secretory duct. ($\times 9,500$)

PLATE 104

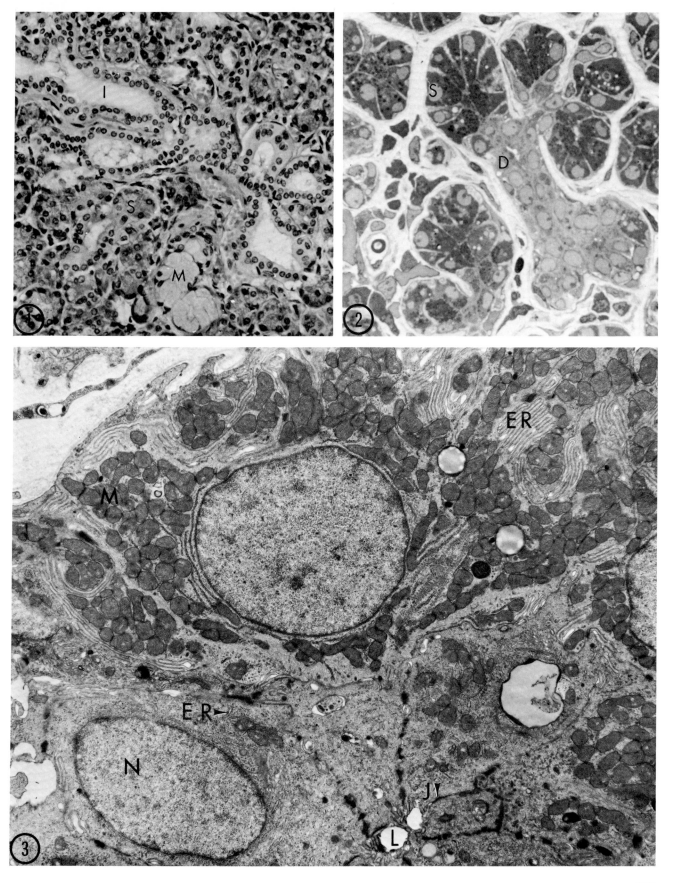

Plate 105 – TASTE BUDS

Figure 1.   Photomicrograph of vallate papilla. Taste buds are most numerous along the walls of the sulci (S) surrounding the vallate papillae but they are also found on fungiform papillae and in pharyngeal mucosa. Taste buds are light-staining oval structures located primarily within the stratified squamous epithelium (SS). Their rounded bases often protrude into the subjacent connective tissue where they contact the afferent nerve fibers. Cells of the taste bud are oriented perpendicular to the lingual surface. ($\times$150)

Figure 2.   Photomicrograph of taste bud. The taste bud is surrounded by stratified squamous epithelium of the lingual mucosa lining the margins of the lingual papillae. A basal lamina (BL) lies between the epithelium and the subjacent connective tissue (CT). Two types of cells comprise the taste buds: light-staining sustentacular cells (Su) and darker-staining neuroepithelial cells (Ne). The neuroepithelial cells terminate at a pit communicating with the lingual surface via a narrow passage called the inner taste pore (IP). Short processes are extended into the pit by the neuroepithelial cells. Sustentacular cells are relatively thick in the middle and taper at each end. Because of the shape of the bud, these elongated cells bend to follow the contour of the taste bud. They intermingle with the neuroepithelial cells and bound the periphery of the taste bud. ($\times$375)

Figure 3.   Electron micrograph of taste bud. The neuroepithelial cells (Ne) are elongated cells terminating at a pit (P) which communicates with the outer lingual surface through the inner taste pore (ITP) bounded by squamous epithelial cells of the lingual mucosa. Sustentacular cells (S) also reach the pit. These cells contain tonofibrils, mitochondria, and, often, lipid bodies (L) in their apical cytoplasm. These are united to the adjacent epithelial cells and the neuroepithelial cells by desmosomes (D). The neuroepithelial cells have a terminal web of tonofibrils in their apical cytoplasm. Portions of this terminal web extend into the interior of taste "hairs," which are irregularly shaped microvilli (Mv). These "hairs" radiate into the pit at the inner pore. Fibrils are also prominent in the rest of the neuroepithelial cell cytoplasm. Isolated membranes of rough-surfaced endoplasmic reticulum, mitochondria and small Golgi vesicles are also present. The apical cytoplasm contains numerous vesicles (V) filled with an electron-dense material. ($\times$11,500)

PLATE 105

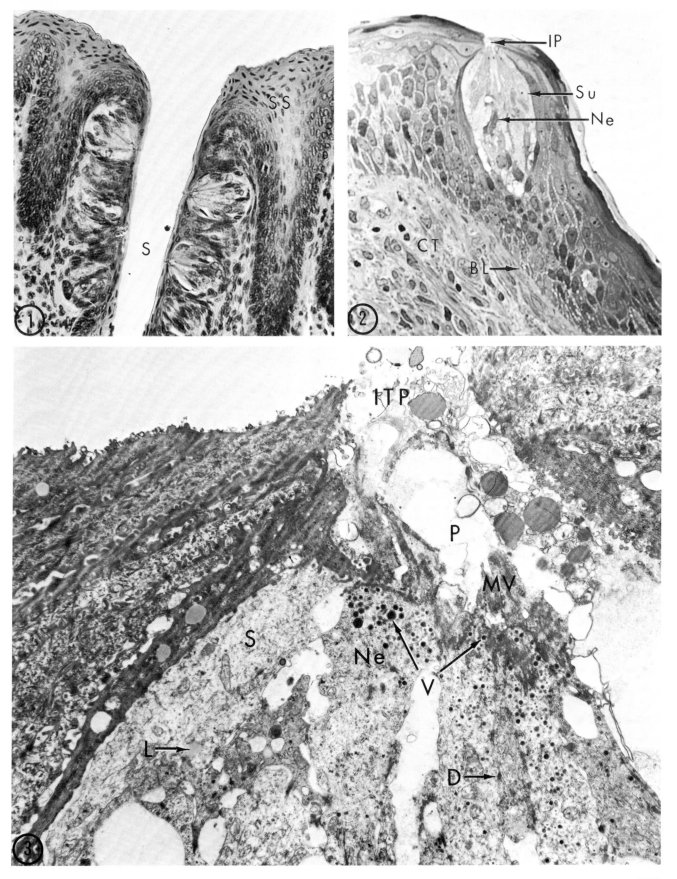

Digestive System

Plate 106 — ESOPHAGUS

Figure 1.   Photomicrograph of esophagus. The wall of the gastrointestinal tube consists of four layers: mucosa, submucosa, muscularis externa, and serosa. The mucous membrane consists of epithelium (E), a connective tissue, lamina propria (LP), and a smooth-muscle muscularis mucosa (MM). The submucosa (SM) of the esophagus is a loose connective tissue in which esophageal glands (EG), vessels and nerves are dispersed. The muscularis externa (ME) consists of skeletal muscle in the upper third and smooth muscle in the lower portion. The epithelium of the esophagus is stratified squamous epithelium. ($\times$60)

Figure 2.   Photomicrograph of esophagus mucosa. The epithelium of the esophagus is stratified squamous. Although connective tissue papillae are present, they are not abundant and do not reduce the thickness of the epithelium significantly. The connective tissue-epithelium interface is relatively smooth. The epithelial cells of the basal layers are basophilic and contain few tonofibrils. Numerous mitoses occur in the basal layers. Cells of the superficial layers are filled with tonofilaments. Nuclei may be seen in some superficial cells while small amounts of keratin may be observed in some regions. This moist epithelium is essentially nonkeratinizing and squamous. The lamina propria (LP) is a thin layer of loose fibrous connective tissue containing ducts of the subjacent esophageal glands in the submucosa. Some mucus-secreting glands may occur in the lower segment of the esophagus. ($\times$375)

Figure 3.   Electron micrograph of esophagus epithelium. The epithelial cells at the surface of nonkeratinizing epithelium may contain nuclei (N) and are generally filled with tonofilaments (Tf). Numerous processes (P) extend into intercellular spaces. Desmosomes (D) unite some of the interdigitating processes of adjacent cells. ($\times$9,000)

PLATE 106

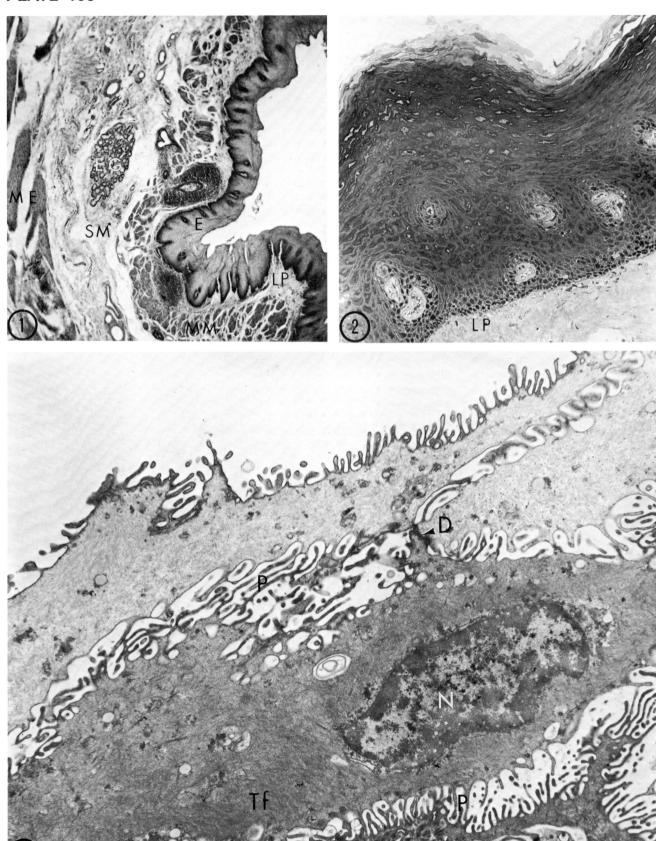

Plate 107 — FUNDIC STOMACH: PARIETAL CELL

Figure 1.   Photomicrograph of mucosa of fundic stomach. The lumen (L) is lined by columnar cells which invaginate to form tubular fundic glands with mucous cells (MN) lining the neck of the glands (FG). (×60)

Figure 2.   Photomicrograph of epon-embedded oblique section of fundic gland. At this level, two cell types are present. The large light-staining cells are the acid-secreting parietal cells. The adjacent epithelial cells are mucus-secreting cells showing clusters of mucous granules. Zymogen-containing chief cells also occur in these glands but are not present at this plane of section. (×375)

Figure 3.   Electron micrograph of parietal cell adjacent to two chief cells. The parietal cell is large and agranular, and its nucleus is eccentrically positioned. The plasma membrane (PM) shows extensive infolding and communicates with intracellular canaliculi (Ca) by means of smooth tubules and vesicles. Mitochondria (M) are numerous. This parietal cell and two chief cells meet at a narrow lumen and are united at this site by junctional complexes (JC). A fibroblast (F) is seen in the lamina propria (LP). (×7,900)

238

PLATE 107

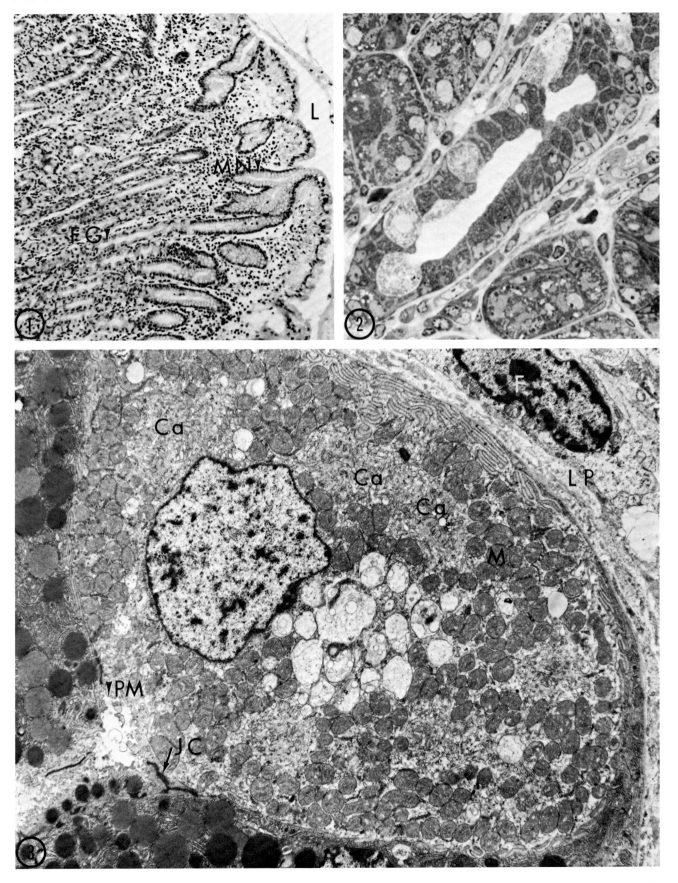

Plate 108 – FUNDIC STOMACH: CHIEF CELL

Figure 1. Photomicrograph of epon-embedded specimen of the mucous neck region of a fundic gland. The neck regions of the fundic glands are relatively short with most of the gland consisting of tubular-shaped clusters of chief and parietal cells. The apices of these mucous neck cells contain clusters of mucous granules (MG). A basal lamina (BL) separates the gland from the adjacent lamina propria (LP). Fibroblasts (F) and plasma cells (P) are present in this figure. ($\times$600)

Figure 2. Photomicrograph of a cross section of the fundic gland. Two cell types may be distinguished. The larger cells are the parietal cells (P) and the smaller cells are the chief cells (C). The apical portions of these cells are filled with zymogen granules. ($\times$375)

Figure 3. Electron micrograph of fundic gland. The central columnar cell is a chief cell. Several large granules of varying size and density, representing different stages of maturation, occupy the apical cytoplasm. Prominent Golgi complexes (G) and small mitochondria (M) as well as membranes of rough endoplasmic reticulum (ER) are distributed between the granules. Membranes of endoplasmic reticulum and mitochondria are also found in the basilar part of the cell with the nucleus (N). The two adjacent cells are parietal cells. Their mitochondria (M) are larger. Few rough ER membranes are present but smooth vesicles and tubules are abundant. A Golgi complex (G) is present but not prominent. Intracellular canals (Ca) with small microvilli are typical of these cells. These canals communicate with the gland lumen and probably represent the site of release of hydrochloric acid. ($\times$12,000)

PLATE 108

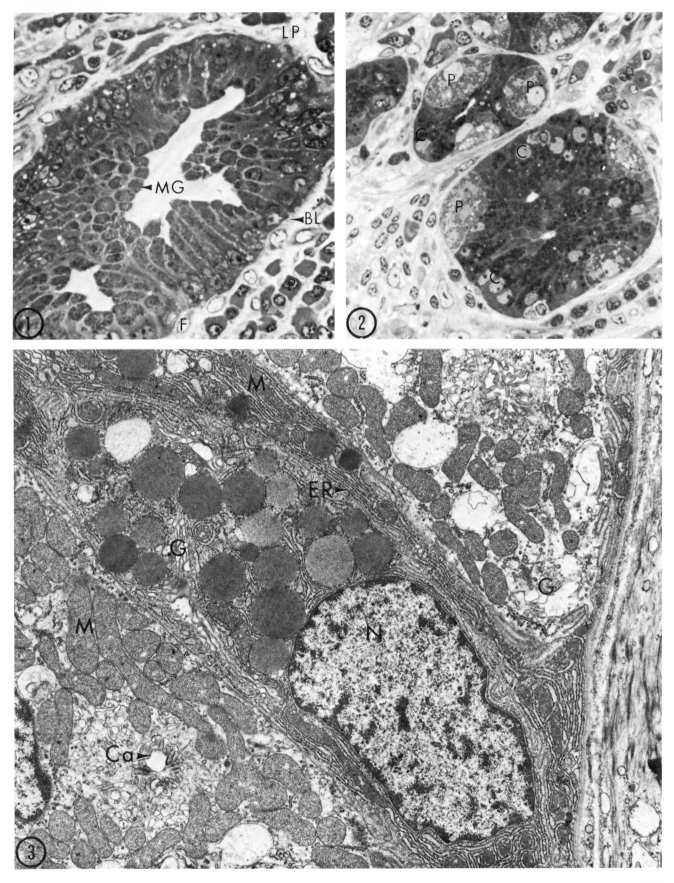

Plate 109 – PYLORIC STOMACH

Figure 1. Photomicrograph of pyloric glands. The mucosa of the stomach consists of columnar mucous surface cells, glandular elements, and a surrounding connective-tissue lamina propria (LP). The gastric pits (P) are continuous with the long necks (N) of the pyloric glands (G). These glands are coiled and consist primarily of mucus-secreting cells. Some argentaffin cells are located between mucous cells. (×60)

Figure 2. Photomicrograph of cross section of epon-embedded pyloric gland. A basal lamina (BL) separates the gland from the surrounding lamina propria (LP). The cells are columnar with nuclei at the basilar end and clusters of mucous inclusions at the distal end. Two argentaffin cells showing a reversal in polarity are indicated by arrows. These cells contain small basophilic granules in the basal-lamina side of the cells. (×375)

Figure 3. Electron micrograph of argentaffin cell surrounded by mucous cells of pyloric gland. The nucleus (N) of the argentaffin cell is centrally placed. Small granules (G) occupy the basal portion of the cytoplasm; they are approximately 0.2 μ in size and homogeneously electron dense. Mitochondria, scattered membranes of rough endoplasmic reticulum and dense inclusions (I) of varying size occupy the cytoplasm. A thin basal lamina (BL) separates the cells from the lamina propria (LP). Mucous inclusions (MI) fill the apices of the adjacent cells. (×7,600)

Figure 4. Electron micrograph of mucous secretory cells. The principal glands of the pylorus produce a mucous secretion. These secretory cells are pyramidal to columnar and have a basal nucleus. The apical ends of the cells have small microvilli (Mv), and are united by tight junctions (TJ). The apical cytoplasm is filled with mucus-secretion vesicles (SV) containing two substances. One substance is electron dense and forms a cap-shaped body contacting the limiting membrane. The second component is less dense and fills most of the vesicle. Rough-surfaced endoplasmic reticulum, small dense mitochondria and a Golgi complex fill the rest of the cytoplasm. (×7,800)

PLATE 109

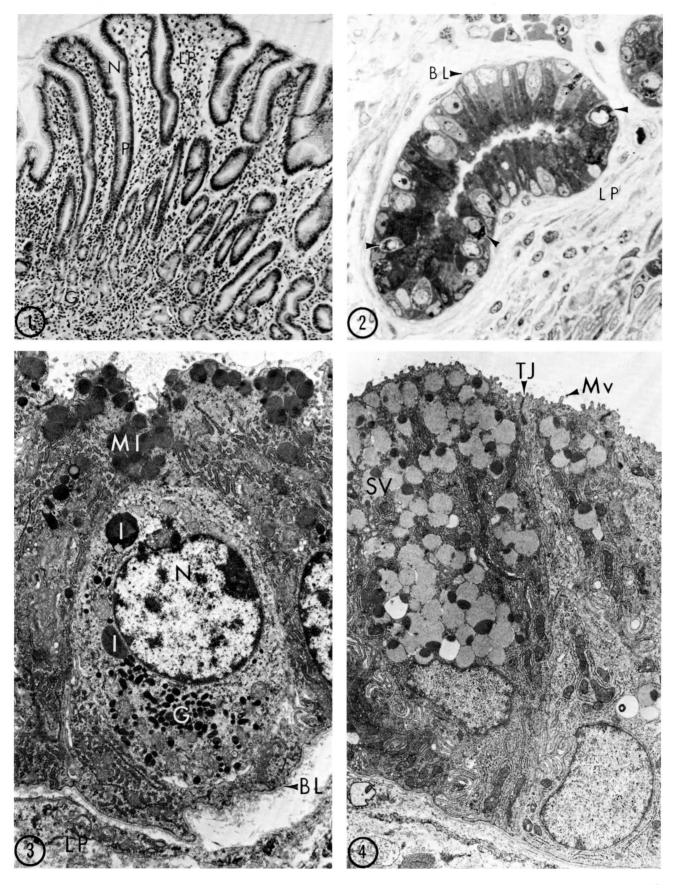

Plate 110 — SMALL INTESTINE: VILLI AND CRYPTS OF LIEBERKÜHN

Figure 1.   Photomicrograph of epon-embedded section of intestinal villus. Villi are finger-like projections with a core of lamina propria (LP) covered with simple columnar epithelium. The surface of these cells shows a striated border (SB) which at higher magnifications proves to be clusters of microvilli. Goblet cells (GC) are interspersed between the regular columnar-lining cells. The epithelial cells develop from dividing cells at the crypts located between villi and move toward the apex of the villus with maturation. (×600)

Figure 2.   Photomicrograph of epon-embedded section of a crypt of Lieberkühn. The cells of the crypts are separated from the subjacent lamina propria (LP) by a thin basal lamina (BL). Capillaries (C) and numerous connective-tissue cells, primarily fibroblasts, occupy this loose fibrous region. In addition to columnar-lining cells and goblet cells, cells with large secretion granules, the Paneth cells (PC), and argentaffin cells are found here. (×575)

Figure 3.   Electron micrograph of Paneth cells from the base of a crypt of Lieberkühn. The lumen of the crypt is just out of view on the left. The base of the cell rests upon the basal lamina (BL) and the nucleus (N) is found in this end of the cell. A nucleolus is prominent. Several large dense and homogeneous secretion granules (SG) occupy the apical end. Membranes of rough endoplasmic reticulum (ER) are extensive. The mitochondria are small and are found throughout the cytoplasm. Golgi lamellae are not prominent in this micrograph but are present and play a significant role in synthesis and organization of these granules. (×11,700)

244

PLATE 116

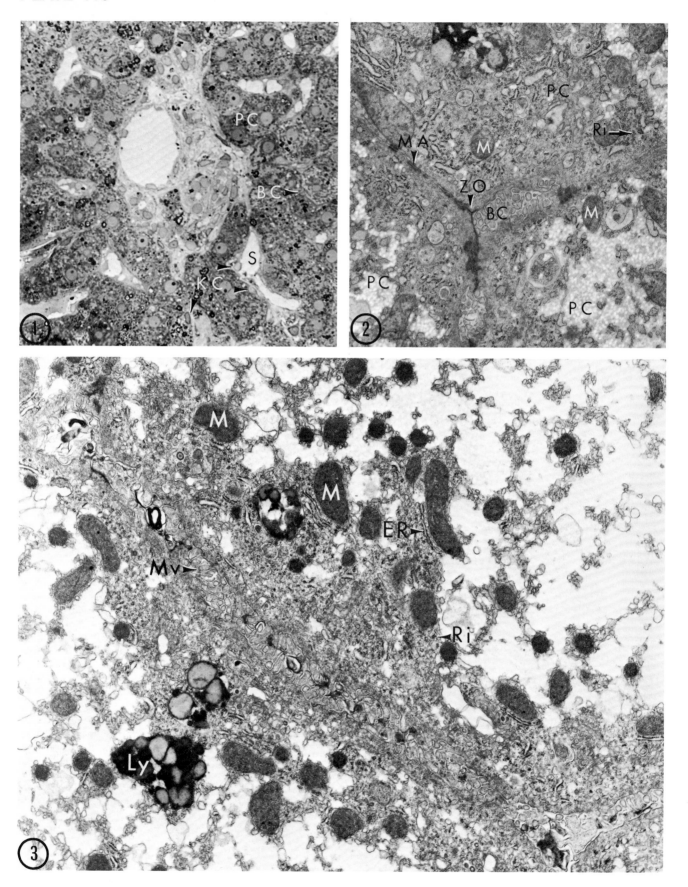

Plate 117 — LIVER

Figure 1. Photomicrograph of liver parenchyma. Arterial and venous blood circulates from vessels in the triads through sinusoids (S) and is collected in the central veins (CV). The sinusoidal spaces between the walls of liver parenchymal cells are lined by Kupffer cells (KC), the liver macrophages which are part of the reticuloendothelial system. (×150)

Figure 2. Photomicrograph of epon-embedded liver. Liver parenchymal cells (PC) serve as the boundary for the sinusoids (S). Flattened basophilic macrophages, the Kupffer cells (KC), serve as a cellular interface between the blood and the parenchymal cells. Materials which pass to and from the parenchymal cells must pass through or between the Kupffer cells. (×375)

Figure 3. Electron micrograph of liver. Three parenchymal cells (PC) surround a sinusoidal space (S). A Kupffer cell (KC) with a dense spindle-shaped nucleus extends thin cytoplasmic processes which approach the parenchymal-cell borders. The plasma membrane of the parenchymal cells has several microvilli (MV) extending toward the Kupffer cell. Some collagen fibrils (Co) occupy the space between the Kupffer cells and the parenchymal-cell microvilli. This intercellular space is called the space of Disse (D). The parenchymal-cell mitochondria (M) are concentrated at the base of the microvilli and are interposed between vesicles containing myelin figures (MF). Membranes of smooth endoplasmic reticulum (SER) are widely distributed throughout the cytoplasm. Electron-dense microbodies (Mb) are also present. (×7,600)

PLATE 117

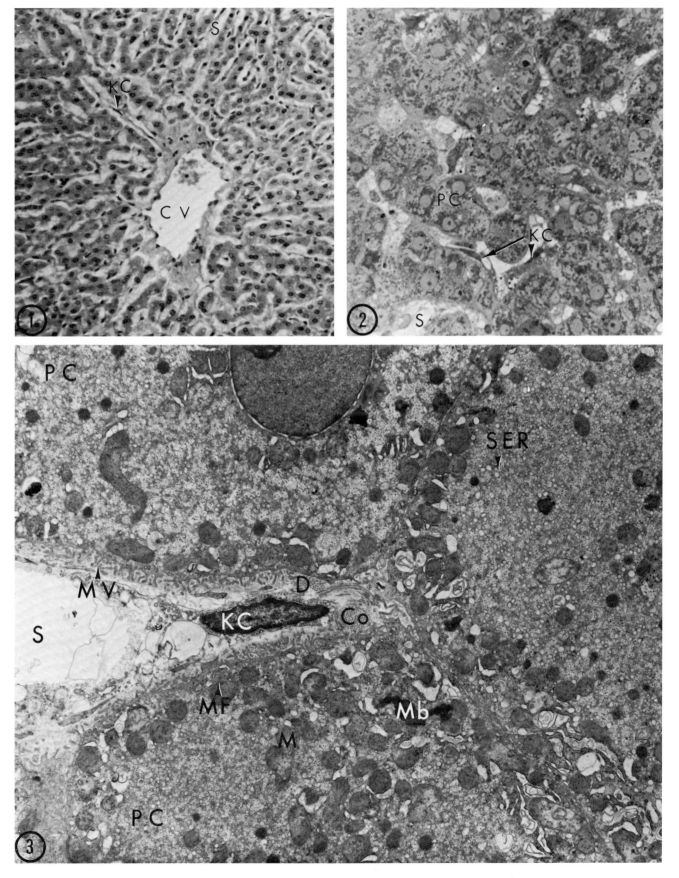

Plate 118 – LIVER

Figure 1.   Photomicrograph of liver triad. The liver lobule is somewhat hexagonal in shape. At the interstices of adjacent lobules, some fibrous connective tissue (CT) is present which usually contains three or more structures: one or more small bile ducts (BD), a terminal of the portal vein (V), and a branch of the hepatic artery (A). These three structures constitute a liver triad. Both blood vessels empty into the sinusoids (S) between the walls of liver parenchymal cells (P). Bile is collected from the canaliculi. (×375)

Figure 2.   Photomicrograph of epon-embedded liver. Triads are located at the margins of liver lobules. In this triad, a branch of the portal vein (V) and three bile ducts (B) are supported by fibrous connective tissue. The branch of the hepatic artery was missed in this section plane. Liver parenchymal cells surround the triad and sheets of these parenchymal cells are separated by sinusoids (S). (×375)

Figure 3.   Electron micrograph of bile duct. The interlobular bile ducts are small and are usually lined with simple cuboidal epithelium. The epithelial cells rest upon a basal lamina (BL) and are supported by collagenous (Co) connective tissue. Unlike that in the pig, this collagen in the human liver triad does not separate individual liver lobules by septa. The cells contain round nuclei (N) located centrally. The lumen (Lu) of the duct is small and irregular. The cytoplasm contains few organelles. (×12,000)

PLATE 118

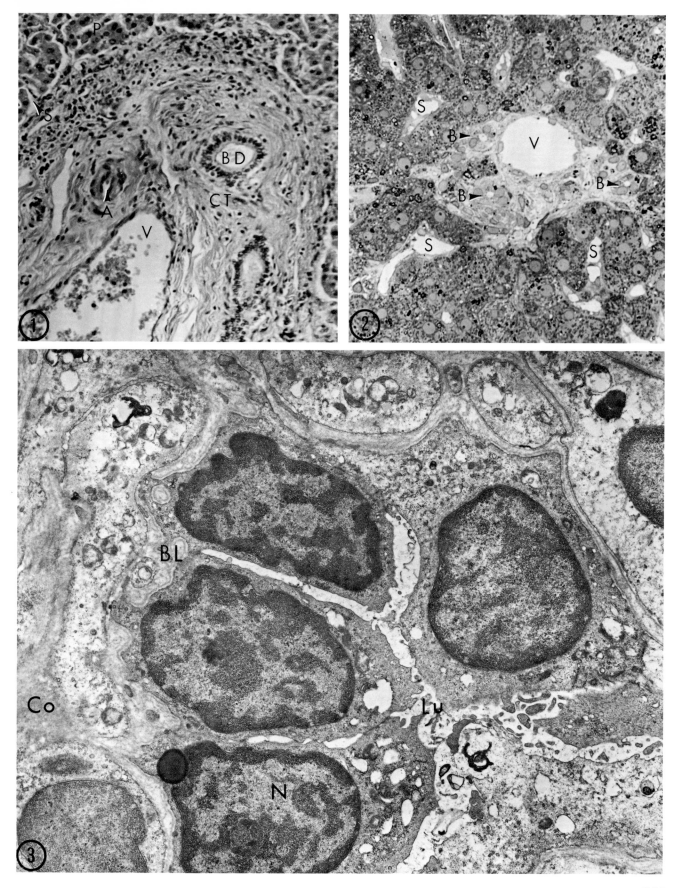

Plate 119 — EXOCRINE PANCREAS

Figure 1. Photomicrograph of H&E-stained section. The pancreas contains both exocrine and endocrine components. The endocrine portion of the gland occurs in isolated groups of cells, the islets of Langerhans (IL), which are surrounded by compound tubuloalveolar exocrine glands. The secretory acini vary in size and shape, ranging from tubular to flask shaped. Sections of exocrine glands rarely show the tubular or alveolar profile, but more often show varying shapes and sizes due to the plane of section. The cells of the secretory units are basophilic and granular, and contain rounded, peripherally disposed nuclei. These empty into ducts, shown in Plate 120. ($\times 150$)

Figure 2. Photomicrograph of epon-embedded section of pancreas. In this field, a light-staining islet of Langerhans (IL) is surrounded by the exocrine portion. The rounded nuclei are at the periphery of the secretory acini (SA). With the enhanced resolution afforded by thin sectioning, definitive clumps of granules are prominent within the cytoplasm. These are the zymogen granules (Z). Ducts (D) are interposed between secretory units. Duct cells are more cuboidal and stain less intensely. ($\times 375$)

Figure 3. Electron micrograph of exocrine portion of pancreas. In this view, the nuclei (N) of three secretory cells are present. The nuclei are rounded, show some condensation of chromatin, and contain one or more nucleoli (Nu). The cells rest upon a basal lamina at one surface and converge upon a small lumen (L) at the opposite cell pole. The cells are narrowed at the luminal surface. Fine microvilli project from the cell surfaces into the lumen. The electron-dense gray material within this lumen is the secretion product. The cytoplasm of these secretory cells contains elongated mitochondria (M), sometimes giving this region a vertically striated appearance. The cytoplasm is filled with abundant membranes of rough endoplasmic reticulum (ER). Rounded dense membrane-bound zymogen granules (Z) are numerous on the luminal side of the cell and are often found in dilated cisternae of the rough endoplasmic reticulum. The zymogen granules are the secretion precursors. The secretory product is protein and explains the prominence of the rough endoplasmic reticulum. A prominent Golgi complex (G) occupies a supranuclear position and is associated with immature zymogen granules of lesser density. ($\times 10,000$)

262

PLATE 119

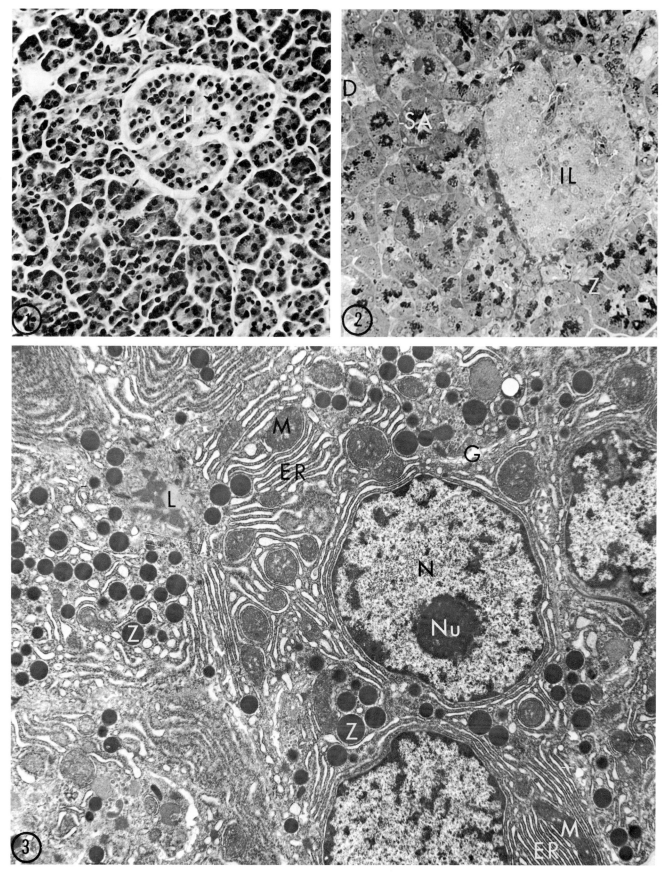

263

Plate 120 — PANCREATIC DUCTS

Figure 1.   Photomicrograph of interlobular duct of pancreas. The lumen (L) is lined with tall columnar epithelium in the larger ducts and low columnar epithelium in the smaller ducts. A layer of connective tissue surrounds the ducts and is continuous with the fibrous septa between lobules. Exocrine secretory units (SU) are clustered in groups around the ducts. The exocrine glands of the pancreas are compound tubuloalveolar. One major duct and an accessory duct 2 to 3 mm wide branch to form interlobar ducts, which in turn branch to form intralobular ducts. (×375)

Figure 2.   Photomicrograph of epon-embedded pancreas. The secretory acini (SU) consist of associated cells which bound a lumen and contain many small basophilic zymogen granules. The contents of the lumina of these units pass through intercalated ducts into the intralobular ducts (D). Cuboidal duct cells are arranged to form a tube one cell thick. The cytoplasm of these cells is clear in comparison to the secretory cells. The nuclei are oval, light staining, and contain an eccentrically positioned nucleolus. (×375)

Figure 3.   Electron micrograph of pancreatic duct. The cuboidal cells are united at tight junctions (TJ), sealing the lining of the lumen (L). Small microvilli (Mv) extend into the lumen from their free surface. The protein-rich secretion appears as a granular precipitate in the lumen. The nucleus (N) with eccentric nucleoli is centrally positioned in the cell. Small mitochondria and tonofilaments are found in the apex and basilar parts of the cell. The basilar plasma membrane (BM) is surrounded by an amorphous basal lamina which adjoins collagen (Co) of the supporting connective-tissue trabeculum. (×12,000)

PLATE 120

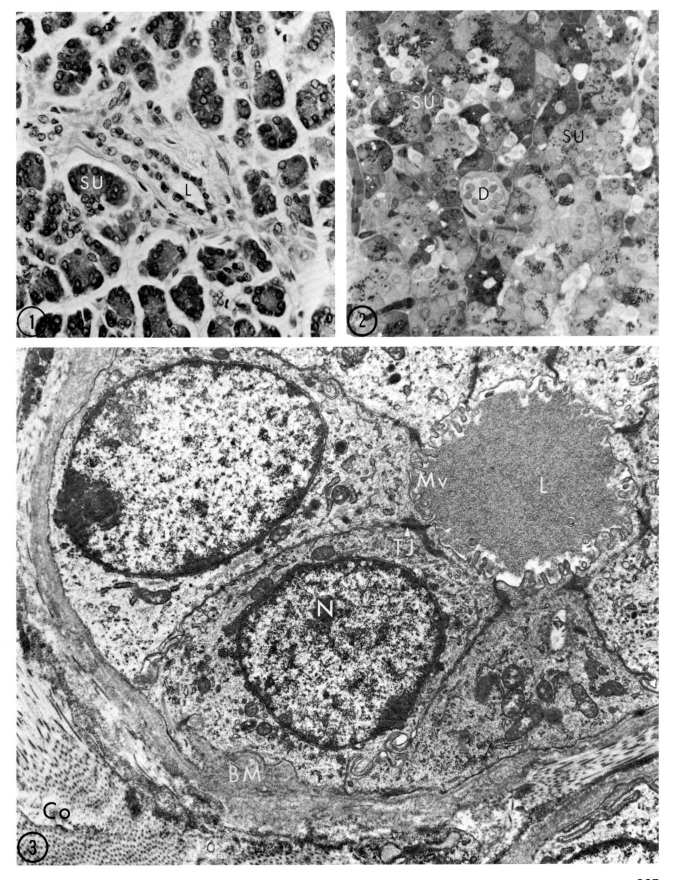

Plate 121 — PANCREAS: CENTROACINAR CELLS

Figure 1.   Photomicrograph of plastic section of exocrine portion of pancreas. The secretory acini (SA) of the glands stain darker and are more irregular in shape than the cells of the ducts (D). Islets (IL) are seen at the bottom and top of the figure. The duct system of the pancreas shows complex branching. Two major ducts enter the pancreas and divide to form a succession of ducts which is first interlobular, then intralobular, and ultimately divided to provide an intercalated duct. Each tubular or flask-shaped secretory acinus receives an intercalated duct. ($\times$350)

Figure 2.   Photomicrograph of plastic section of exocrine pancreas. Each of the darker secretory cells contains basophilic electron-dense zymogen granules. Intercalated ducts are seen both outside the acini and continuous with the secretory units. Some of these duct cells extend into the lumen of the secretory acini and are called centroacinar cells (Ca). ($\times$650)

Figure 3.   Electron micrograph of secretory acinus in which both secretory cells and duct cells comprise the outer limits of the lumen (L). The secretory cells contain the characteristic zymogen granules (Z) and an extensive rough endoplasmic reticulum (ER). Both secretory and duct cells extend microvilli into the lumen, which contains the protein secretion. The duct cells (CA) have rounded nuclei, less osmophilic cytoplasm, and fewer organelles. The mitochondria (M) of these cells are small and tubular. The entire acinus, including both secretory cells and centroacinar cells, is surrounded by the basal lamina (B) which is continuous with the basal lamina of the intercalated ducts. ($\times$8,700)

266

PLATE 121

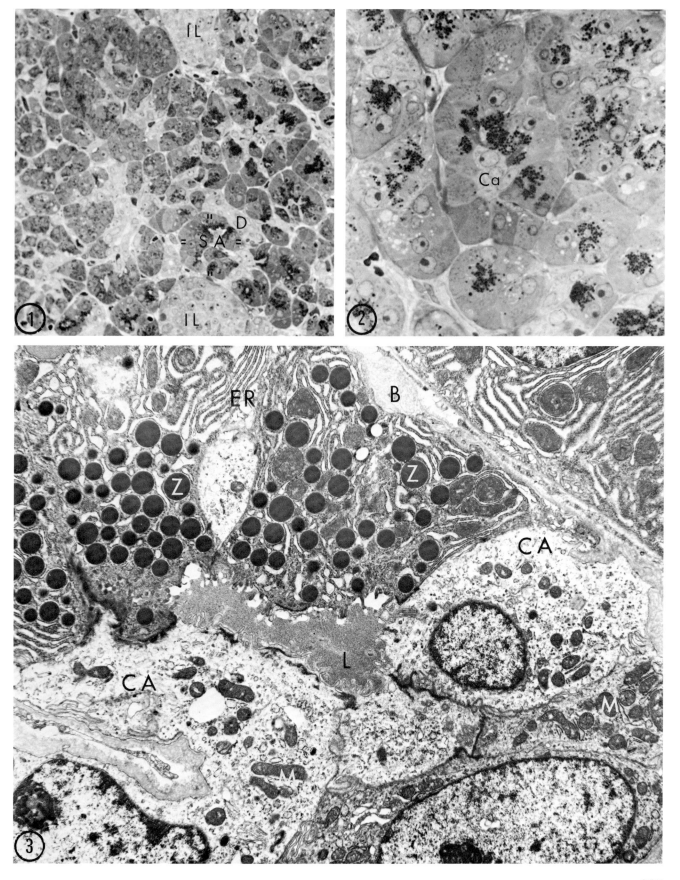

PLATE 127

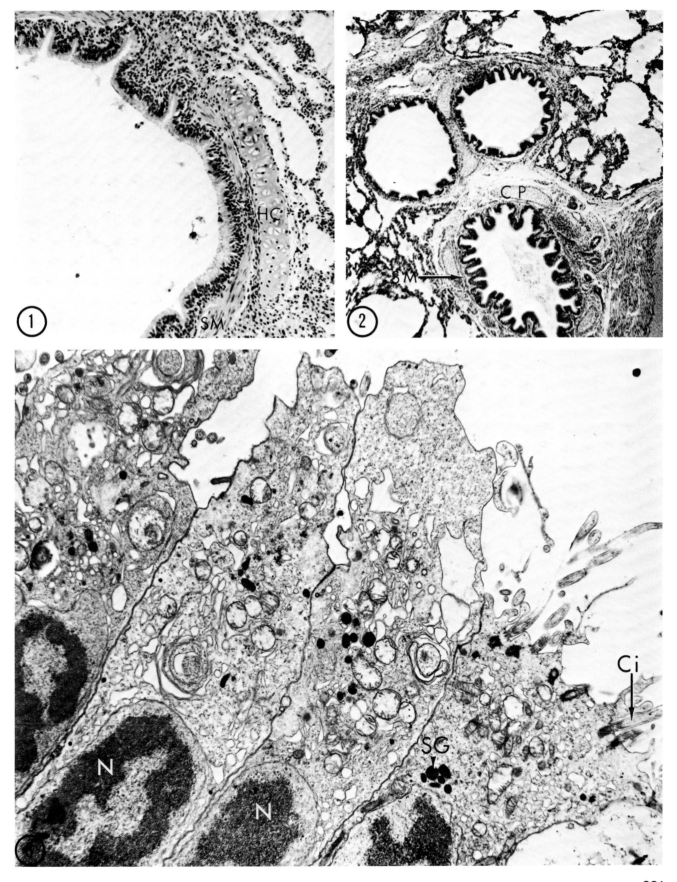

Plate 128 – RESPIRATORY BRONCHIOLE

Figure 1. Photomicrograph of respiratory bronchiole. These structures connect the conducting division of the respiratory system with the true respiratory division where gas exchange occurs between blood vessels and alveolar spaces. The respiratory bronchiole (RB) consists of simple cuboidal epithelium supported by smooth muscle fibers (SM) and fibrous connective tissue. The cuboidal epithelium of the respiratory bronchiole is continuous with the simple squamous epithelium of the alveolar sacs (AS) and alveolar ducts. Respiratory bronchioles are continuous proximally with the terminal bronchioles, which have a columnar epithelium and a more muscular wall. (×150)

Figure 2. Photomicrograph of epon-embedded respiratory bronchiole. The epithelium at the right of the figure lines a terminal bronchiole (TB). This epithelium is simple ciliated columnar. After reduction in height it becomes the simple cuboidal epithelium of the respiratory bronchiole (RB). It is continuous with the squamous epithelium lining the alveolar sacs (AS). A fibrous stroma with some smooth muscle fibers supports the bronchiole epithelium. Macrophages (M) containing numerous small dense inclusions are found in the supporting tissue. These are called clasmatocytes or dust cells in the lung. (×375)

Figure 3. Electron micrograph of respiratory bronchiole. The epithelium of the respiratory bronchiole is simple cuboidal epithelium becoming thin as it terminates at the alveolar duct. The cells rest upon a basal lamina and are supported by a thin fibrous connective-tissue stroma in which both collagen and elastic (E) fibers are dispersed. Adjacent cells are united at their lateral surface by desmosomes (D). Tight junctions are found at the apical margins. Numerous microvilli project a short distance into the air passageway. The cytoplasm is filled with numerous free ribosomes and has several membranes of rough-surfaced endoplasmic reticulum. A Golgi complex (G) is present and small membrane-limited electron-dense vesicles (V) are located in the apical cytoplasm. The plasma membrane is crowded with pinocytotic vesicles. This cell appears to be equipped for secretion. (×8,900)

Figure 4. Electron micrograph of dust cell. Macrophages in the lung receive particulate matter ingested and subsequently discharged by lining cells. The cells are located within the supporting stroma of the lung. The nuclei (N) are irregular in shape and have a condensed chromatin pattern. The cytoplasm contains a large Golgi complex (G). Mitochondria are large, tubular and widely distributed. A few lysosomes are present. Membrane-limited phagocytized inclusions (PI) are seen at the cell periphery and deep within the cytoplasm. (×12,700)

PLATE 128

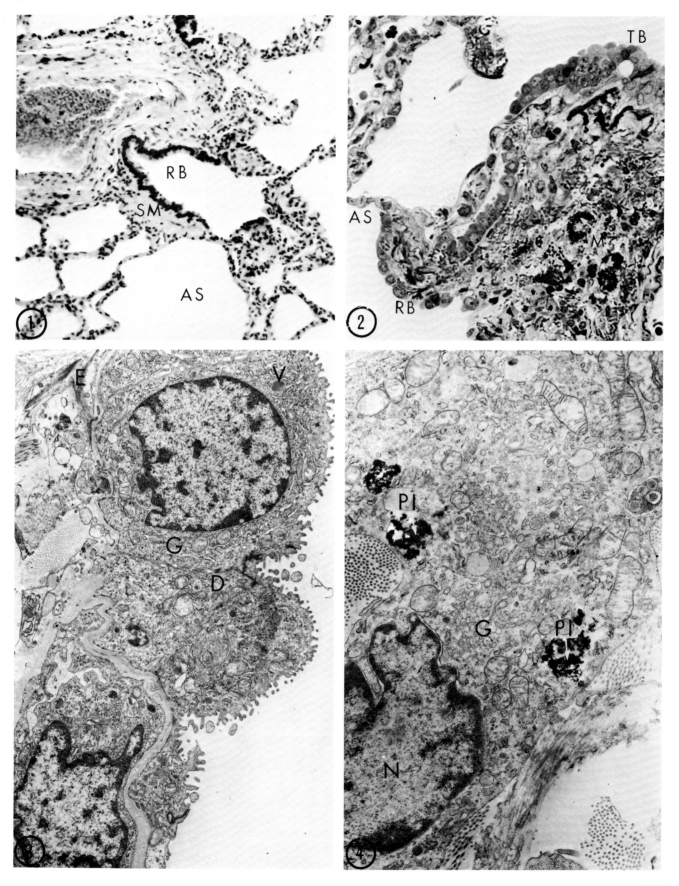

Plate 129 — LUNG

Figure 1.   Photomicrograph of alveolar sacs and respiratory bronchioles. Respiratory bronchioles are the connecting structures between the conducting and active respiratory divisions of this system. The epithelium of the respiratory bronchiole is simple cuboidal and is continuous with the simple squamous epithelium of the alveoli. Larger blood vessels (BV) may be found in the connective tissue of these bronchioles. The lumen of the respiratory bronchiole (B) empties into an elongated space, the alveolar duct (AD), the lumen of which is contiguous with the lumen of the alveolar sacs (AS). ($\times$60)

Figure 2.   Photomicrograph of epon-embedded section of alveolar wall. Two types of cells comprise the epithelial lining of the alveoli. Flat, simple squamous epithelial cells (EC) alternate randomly with secretory epithelial cells (SC). These cells have secretory granules within their cytoplasm. If they are a part of the epithelial lining, they are termed Type I cells. The large cells released into the air spaces are termed Type II cells (T2). ($\times$375)

Figure 3.   Electron micrograph of alveolar wall. A Type I epithelial cell (TI) is barely connected to a lining epithelial cell at the arrow. Numerous lamellated secretion bodies (SB) are distributed in the cytoplasm. These are believed to contain phospholipid which acts as a surfactant when released to the alveolar space. Microvilli (Mv) are usually limited to the cell surface exposed to air but extend to more of the cell surface when it detaches from the true epithelial lining. The mitochondria (M) are spherical and almost devoid of cristae. Collagen fibers (Co) separate the basal lamina of the epithelial cells from the basal lamina surrounding a capillary (C). ($\times$11,600)

PLATE 129

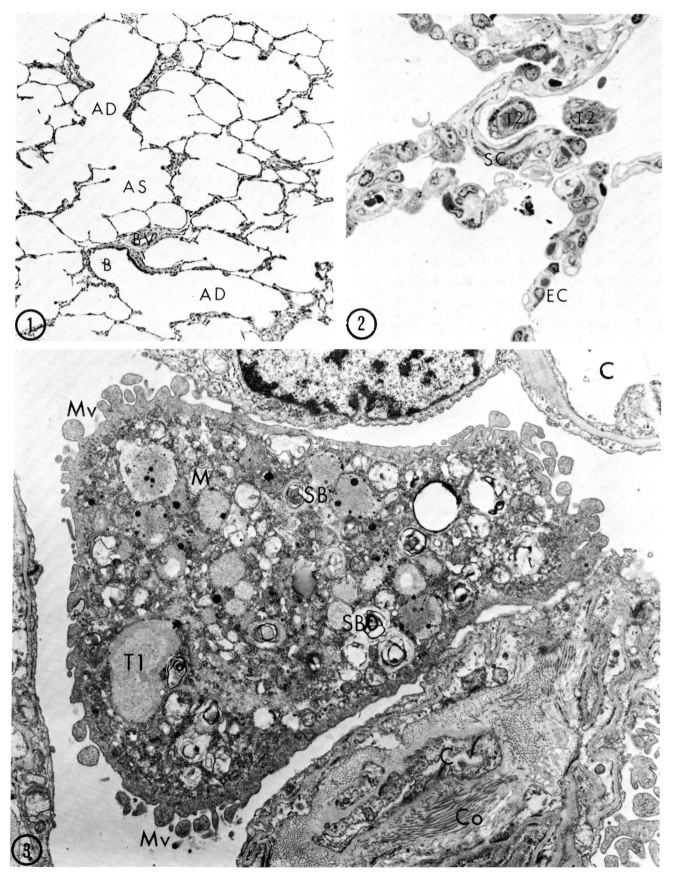

Urinary System

Plate 130 – KIDNEY: GENERAL STRUCTURE

Figure 1. Photomicrograph of kidney cortex. The cortex of the kidney consists of nephrons and associated blood vessels and collecting ducts. The nephron is the functional unit of the kidney and consists of a glomerulus, a renal capsule, and renal tubules. Some parts of the renal tubules extend into the kidney medulla but all of the glomeruli (G) are in the cortex. The human kidney has 10 to 18 lobes. Each lobe consists of a pyramid of medullary tubules, together with a base of cortical structures. Lobes are divided into functional regions called lobules, regions of lobes in which the nephrons drain into a common collecting tube. Groups of collecting ducts serve as cores of lobules and these regions are called medullary rays (MR). The renal tubules served by the ducts of the medullary rays follow a tortuous course; thus this surrounding cortical tissue is called the cortical labyrinth (CL). (×60)

Figure 2. Photomicrograph of renal corpuscle. The renal corpuscle consists of glomerulus (G) and a surrounding renal capsule. The capsule is termed the parietal layer of Bowman's capsule (BC). Cells of this capsule are continuous with the epithelial cells, the podocytes, investing the glomerular capillaries (Ca). The urinary space (US) between Bowman's capsule and podocyte receives the glomerular filtrate. The glomerular filtrate is emptied into the proximal convoluted tubules (PC); reabsorption of water, glucose, etc., occurs in these and the succeeding tubules of the nephron. Another tubule of the nephron characteristically found near the renal corpuscle is the distal convoluting tubule (DC), which ultimately empties urine into the collecting ducts.

The capillaries of the glomeruli receive blood from afferent arterioles (AA) and empty into efferent arterioles. (×375)

Figure 3. Electron micrograph of renal corpuscle. The parietal layer of Bowman's capsule (PBC) consists of a layer of simple squamous epithelium resting upon a basal lamina (BL). A capillary (C) in the glomerulus consists of simple squamous endothelial cells with very thin cytoplasm. Numerous fenestrae (arrows) are seen in the endothelial cells, which rest upon a basal lamina (BL). The opposite surface of this basal lamina is covered intermittently by foot processes of podocytes which constitute the visceral layer of Bowman's capsule. Capillary plasma passes through the endothelial cell fenestra, through the basal lamina, between foot processes, into the urinary space (US). The fluid in this space is the glomerular filtrate. (×11,300)

PLATE 130

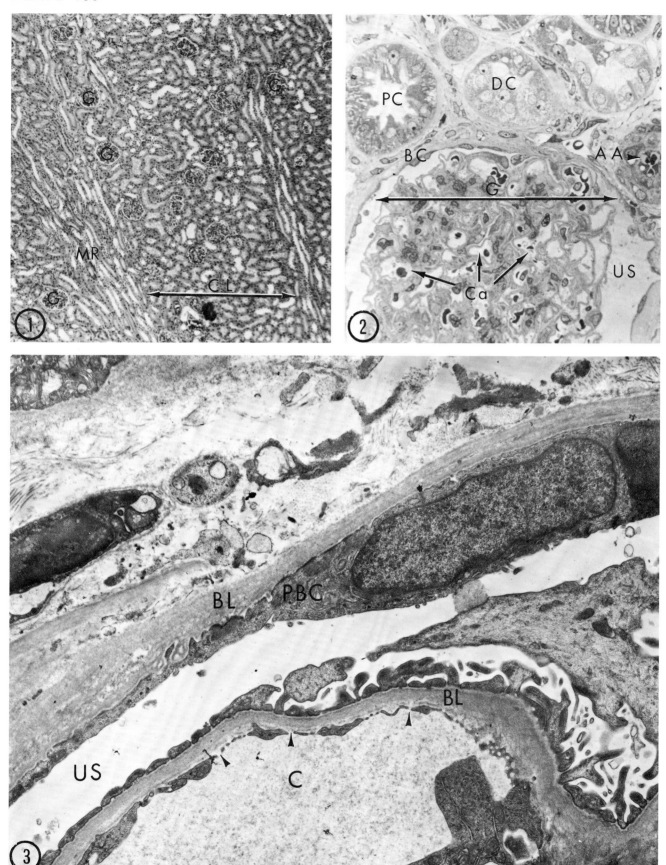

Plate 131 — KIDNEY: MESANGIAL CELL

Figure 1. Electron micrograph of mesangial cell. As glomerular capillaries branch from the afferent artery and converge on the efferent artery, the diverging and converging vessels are closely approximated. These "stalk" areas between adjacent capillaries are not opposed by podocytes; hence, the basal lamina contributed by the secretory activity of the podocytes is not present. These sites are occupied by special cells, the mesangial cells. Mesangial cells (MC) contribute to the formation of an incomplete basal lamina (IBL) supporting the vessels in these areas. The mesangial cell is separated from a capillary (Ca) by the incompletely formed basal lamina. Mesangial cells resemble pericytes but they also contain granules (JG) similar to those found in the juxtaglomerular cells of the afferent arteriole. Granules of juxtaglomerular cells are believed to secrete renin, a substance causing the release of angiotensin II and an increased output of aldosterone by the adrenal cortex. Granules in the mesangial cells, like those in JG cells, are of varying size and density and are irregular in shape.

Mesangial cells are stellate shaped, have a large granular nucleus, and often extend cytoplasmic processes (CP) between segments of basal lamina to terminate directly on the endothelial cells (EC). Phagocytic vesicles, rough-surfaced endoplasmic reticulum, free ribosomes, and a Golgi complex occupy the cytoplasm. Small intracellular filaments are prominent in the processes.

Lateral to the mesangial cell and its related capillaries, foot processes (FP) and major processes (MP) of podocytes are seen between true continuous basal lamellae (BL). Fenestrated endothelial cells of adjacent capillaries line these basal lamellae on the opposite surface. (×17,800)

PLATE 131

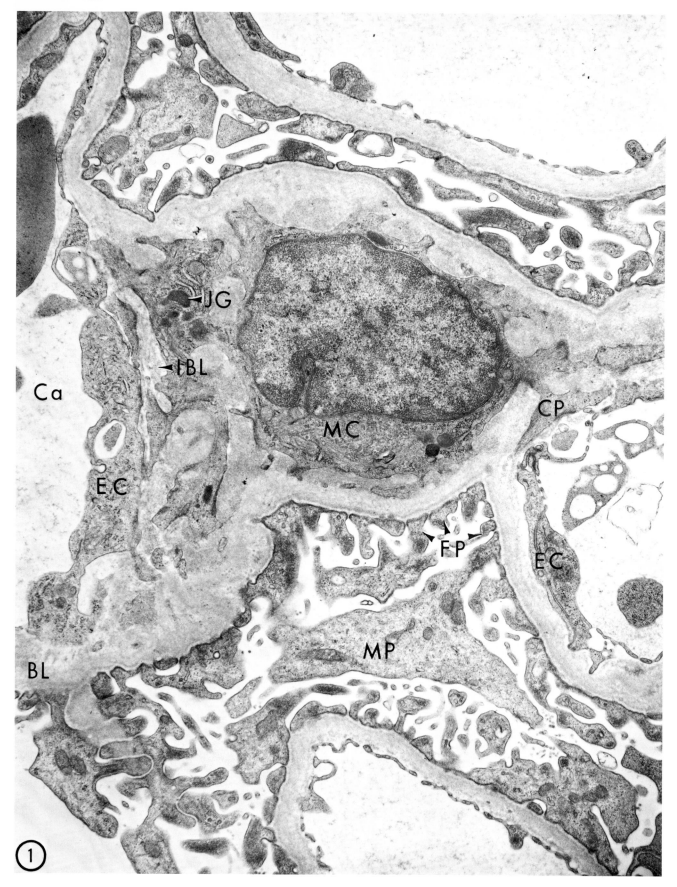

①

Plate 132 — KIDNEY: PODOCYTE

Figure 1. Electron micrograph of glomerulus. The basal lamina (BL) is the true filtration barrier of the glomerulus. The plasma of the capillary (C) has access to the substance of the basal lamina via the fenestrae (F) of the capillary endothelial cell. Large molecules such as albumin do not ordinarily pass through this lamina but are kept as plasma constituents. Water, electrolytes, and smaller organic molecules pass through the lamina and enter the space between foot processes (FP) of the podocyte. Podocytes (P) are squamous epithelial cells lining the urinary space. These cells have a large nucleus (N), a nucleolus and large processes that bifurcate to form foot processes. The cytoplasm of these cells contains few organelles. (×14,000)

Figure 2. Electron micrograph of glomerulus. The capillaries (C) of the glomerulus originate from larger vessels at the glomerular stalk. The capillaries follow a tortuous course and ultimately end in larger vessels emptying into the efferent arteriole. This arrangement is especially suitable for the extrusion of fluid and solutes from the glomerular capillary, as a high hydrostatic pressure is maintained along its entire length. The cytoplasm of the endothelial cells is attenuated with the exception of the cytoplasm surrounding the endothelial cell nucleus. Numerous pores (fenestrae) occur in these cells, providing a route for the passage of plasma to the functional filtration barrier, the basal lamina (BL). Foot processes (FP) of podocytes line the urinary space (US) on the opposite surface of the basal lamina. Foot processes are terminations of major processes (MP) of podocytes. Because of the varying course of the capillaries, several section planes may be obtained in one glomerular area. The capillary on the right was sectioned in such a plane that the fenestrae of the endothelial cells are seen in a surface view. They appear as round to oval pores limited by plasma membrane of the endothelial cell. (×14,000)

PLATE 132

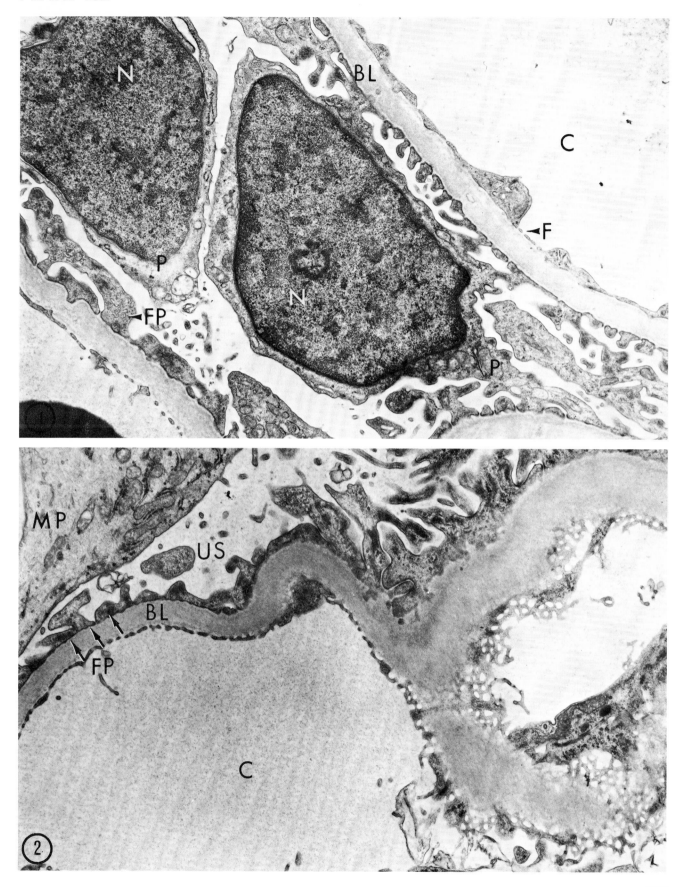

Plate 133 – KIDNEY: PROXIMAL CONVOLUTING TUBULE

Figure 1. Photomicrograph of renal corpuscle and surrounding tissue. The glomerular filtrate, produced in the renal corpuscle (RC), empties into the proximal convoluted tubule (PCT). This tubule is 10 to 20 mm in length with a diameter of 50 to 70 μ. The tubule follows a looped tortuous course near the renal corpuscle, hence the name convoluted tubule. The tubes then straighten and follow the course of the medullary rays toward the medulla where they terminate in loops of Henle. The lining cells have round nuclei positioned at the cell base adjacent to the basal lamina. The lumen surface of these cells is irregular and shows a striated appearance or brush border consisting of microvilli. The cytoplasm of these cells is more granular and more extensive than the cytoplasm of cells of distal convoluting tubules. ($\times$150)

Figure 2. Photomicrograph of renal cortex. A renal corpuscle (RC) is bounded by Bowman's capsule (BC). An afferent arteriole (AA) lies just outside this capsule and supplies blood to the glomerular capillaries (GC). Proximal convoluted tubules (PC) occur in several forms as the plane of section cuts through the twisting tubules in different positions. The cells are pyramidal in shape, possessing a broad base and a tapering apical portion. Their brush border (BB) appears as a thick light-staining band lining the narrow lumen. Peritubular capillaries (PTC) occupy the intertubular space. ($\times$375)

Figure 3. Electron micrograph of proximal convoluting tubule. The lumen (Lu) is bounded by pyramidal-shaped cells possessing a brush border, a series of microvilli (Mv) about 1 μ long. The nucleus is round, and occupies the basal part of the cell. The adjacent plasma membrane rests upon a basal lamina (BL). Adjacent cells are bound by desmosomes (D) and tight junctions (TJ) unite adjacent cells near their apical free surface. The cytoplasm has an abundance of free ribosomes (Ri), a few membranes of rough-surfaced endoplasmic reticulum, and large, round, widely distributed mitochondria (M). A small Golgi complex (G) is present. The cells have a wide basal portion, so cross sections of the tubules show widely separated nuclei. The microvilli are lost as the proximal tubules descend toward Henle's loop. ($\times$11,400)

PLATE 133

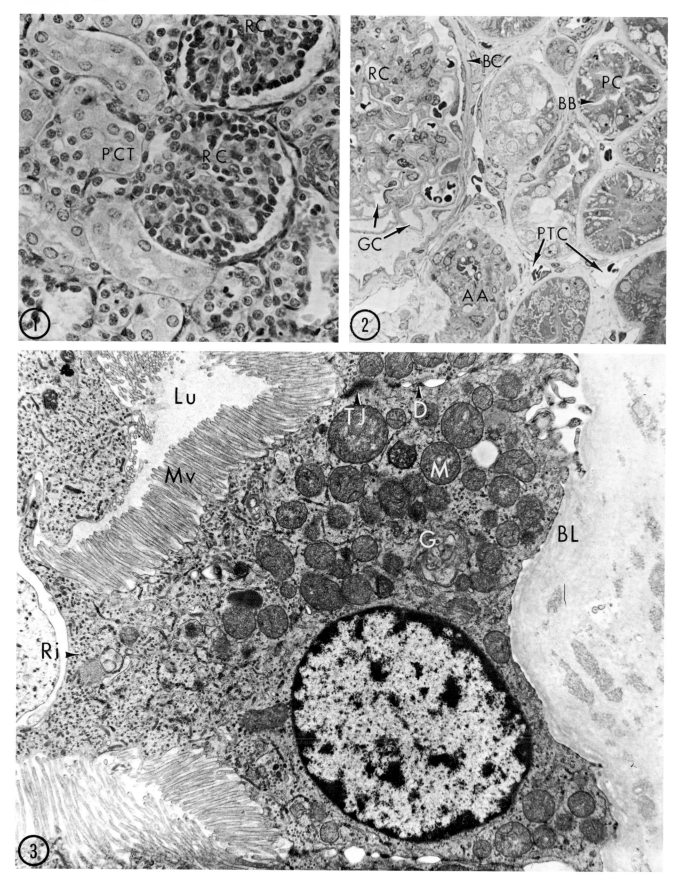

Plate 134 — KIDNEY: DISTAL CONVOLUTING TUBULE

Figure 1.	Photomicrograph of kidney cortex. Two renal corpuscles (Gl) are surrounded by sections of proximal and distal convoluting tubules. The proximal tubules (PT) are longer than the distal tubules (DT), so sections of the former are more numerous in any field. Proximal tubules have a larger outer diameter than distal tubules. The distal tubules may have a larger lumen diameter, as the cuboidal cells of distal tubules are smaller and do not have a brush border. Because of their small cell size, the small round nuclei of the distal tubules are often closer together. (×150)

Figure 2.	Photomicrograph of epon-embedded kidney tubules. The cells of the proximal tubules (PT) are low columnar and show a definitive and light-staining striated lumen surface. This surface consists of microvilli and is referred to as the brush border (BB). A basal lamina (BL) surrounds this and the adjacent distal convoluted tubule (DT). The latter has a cuboidal type of epithelium with round, centrally placed nuclei. One or more small nucleoli may be seen. Microvilli are not prominent. The basilar part of the cells contains elongated mitochondria. Capillaries are present in the intertubular alveolar tissue. (×375)

Figure 3.	Electron micrograph of distal convoluting tubule. The lumen (L) of the distal tubule is bounded by cuboidal cells resting upon a basal lamina (BL). Capillaries (C) are adjacent to the lamina and are supported by a loose collagenous (Co) matrix. The nuclei (N) are round and of even density. The lumen surface shows a few small microvilli (Vi). Tight junctions (TJ) are found at the apical junction of contiguous cells. The membranes of contiguous cells interdigitate by complex folds (F). The basilar membrane also shows pronounced infolding, producing membrane-limited segments of basal cytoplasm called basal processes (BP). Electron-dense elongated mitochondria occupy these basal processes. Processes of adjacent contiguous cells may interdigitate at the basal lamina. A prominent Golgi complex (GC) and numerous small vesicles (Ve) are apically positioned in each cell. Small vesicles also form at the basilar membrane. One segment of distal tubules adheres to the Bowman's capsule of the nephron at the glomerular root; at this site the nuclei of the distal cells are closer together, forming the macula densa. (×11,700)

PLATE 134

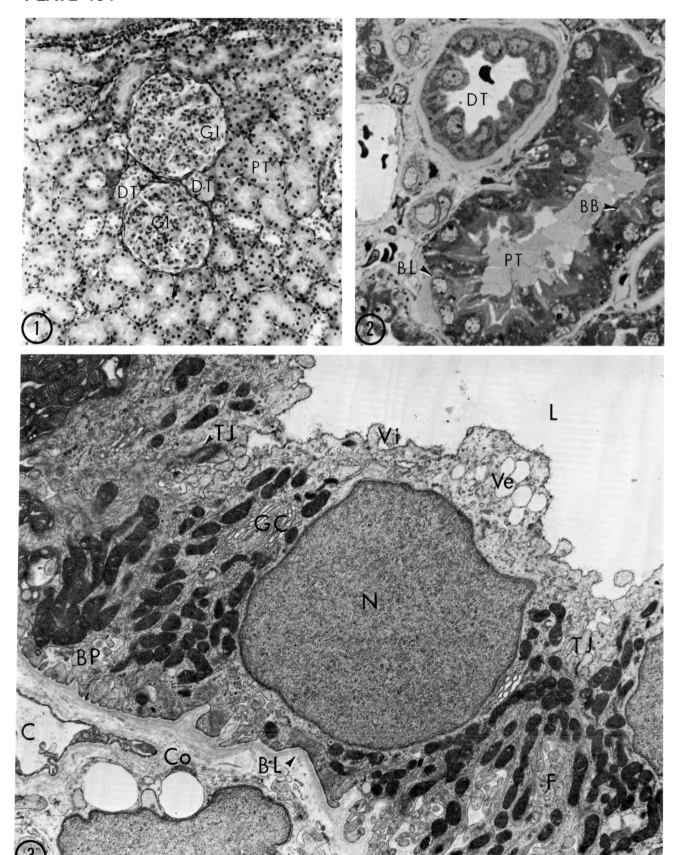

Plate 135 – KIDNEY: MEDULLA

Figure 1.   Photomicrograph of kidney medulla. The main medullary mass consists of 8 to 20 medullary pyramids. The pyramid base contacts the cortex and the apex projects into a minor calyx. The medulla contains no glomeruli but consists of ascending and descending limbs (L) and thin segments (T) of nephrons, collecting ducts (D) and peritubular capillaries. (×70)

Figure 2.   Photomicrograph of medullary ray and adjacent cortical labyrinth. Portions of the medulla appear to project into the cortex. This appearance of medullary rays in the cortex is due to the presence of collecting ducts and the medullary part of nephrons with glomeruli situated close to the kidney capsule. The tubules of these outer glomeruli are not long enough to reach the medulla proper. Thus, thin-walled segments (TS) may be seen adjacent to proximal (P) and distal convoluting tubules (DCT). Blood vessels (BV) occupy the inter-tubular spaces. (×400)

Figure 3.   Electron micrograph of ascending limb of nephron. The tubular portion of the nephron is composed of: (1) the proximal convoluted tubule; (2) straight segment of the proximal tubule; (3) proximal segment of Henle's loop; (4) thin segment of Henle's loop; (5) thick distal segment of Henle's loop; (6) ascending segment; and (7) distal convoluting tubule. The latter empties into a collecting duct which is not considered a part of the nephron. The thin segment of Henle's loop consists of squamous epithelial cells. The nuclei of these cells bulge into the lumen. Most of the cytoplasm is in the perinuclear region. Few organelles are seen within these cells. At the union of the thin segment and the ascending limb seen in this figure, the cells are flat but the cytoplasm is not as attenuated as in the thin segment. The nuclei (N) are oval. A few mitochondria, free ribosomes and some rough-surfaced endoplasmic reticulum are present. Occa-sional small microvilli (Mv) project into the lumen (Lu) filled with precipitated protein from the urine. Adjacent epithelial cells are joined by desmosomes. Tight junctions (TJ) unite the plasma membranes as they approach the lumen. A basal lamina (BL) and loose collagenous connective tissue surround the tubule. (×14,000)

298

PLATE 135

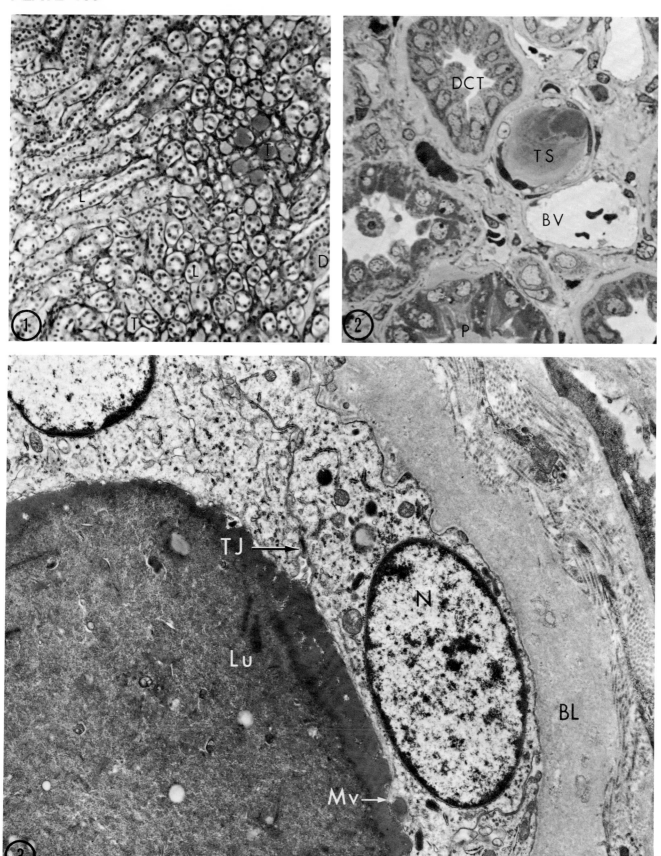

Plate 136 — URETER

Figure 1.   Photomicrograph of ureter. The wall of the ureters consists of a mucosa (Mu), muscularis (Ms) and adventitia (Ad). The lumen is star shaped, as the mucosal epithelium has regular folds with connective-tissue cores. Only part of the lumen and a few folds are seen at this magnification. Transitional epithelium and connective tissue form the mucosa. The muscularis consists of smooth-muscle fibers arranged in three layers. Fibers of the middle layer follow a circular direction while the inner and outer fiber layers follow a longitudinal course. The adventitia is fibrous connective tissue. (×150)

Figure 2.   Photomicrograph of ureter mucosa. The epithelium of the ureter is transitional. The basal lamina (BL) is relatively straight. Cells of the basilar layers are cuboidal while cells of the superficial layers are elongated. The large pear-shaped surface cells typical of transitional epithelium of the urinary bladder are not common. A fibrous lamina propria (LP) separates the epithelium from the surrounding muscularis. (×375)

Figure 3.   Electron micrograph of epithelial cells of ureter. The free surfaces of these cells have numerous small microvilli (Mv). A tight junction (TJ) is seen at the lateral junction of cell apices. Opposing plasma membranes are held close in the superficial cell layers, but deeper cells are more widely separated. Numerous cell processes (CP) of contiguous cells are extended into the intercellular spaces. Free ribosomes (Ri) are the most prominent cytoplasmic feature. The nuclei are rounded with evenly dispersed chromatin. (×9,200)

300

PLATE 136

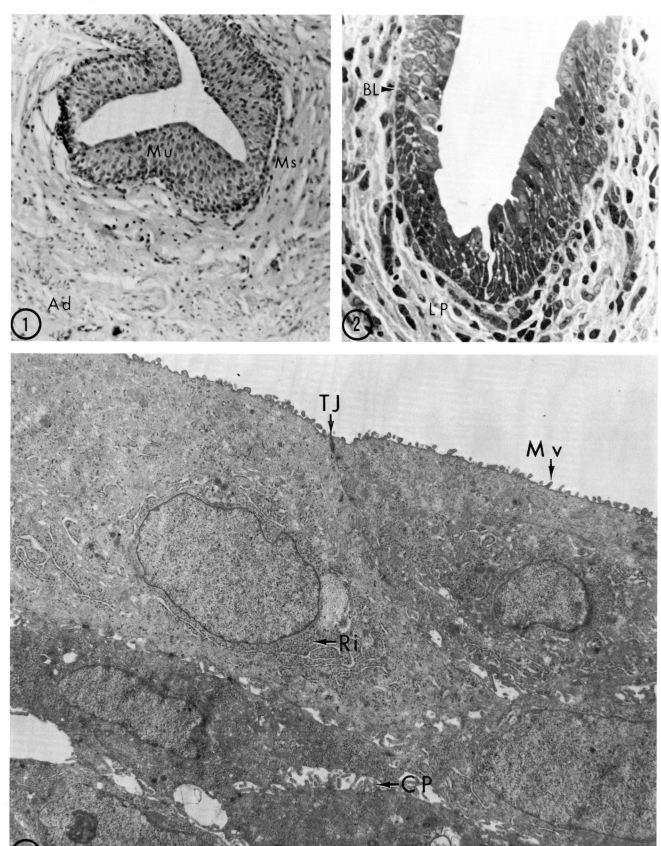

PLATE 142

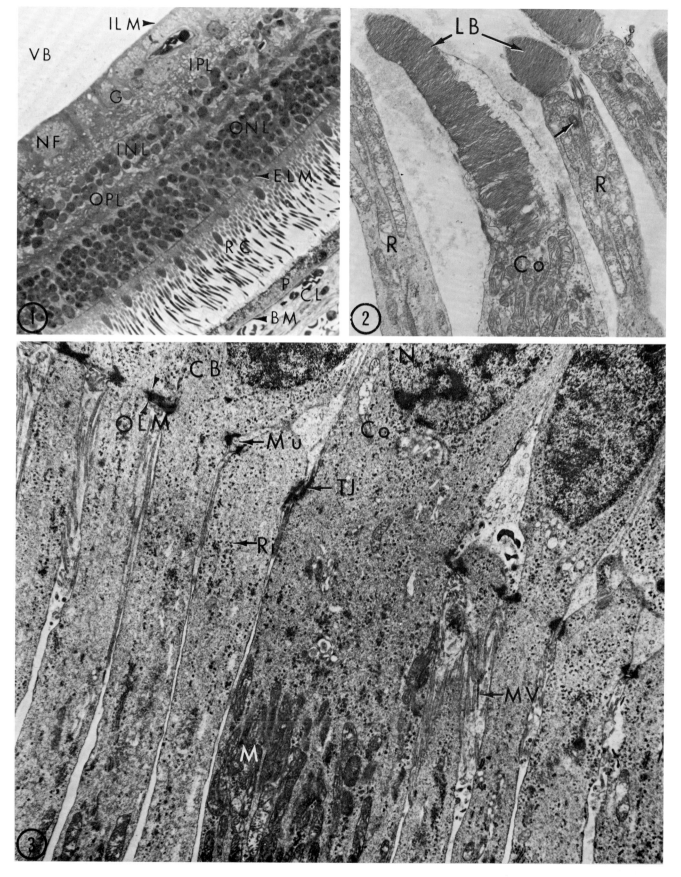

Plate 143 — RETINA

Figure 1. Electron micrograph of rods. The light-sensitive elements of the retina, the outer rod segment, are situated on the distal ends of rods and cones. These structures have a lamellar arrangement of membranes invested in a pocket of plasma membrane (P). Each lamellated structure is attached to the main cell body by a stalk which closely resembles a cilium. A basal body (BB) or centriole is located at the apex of the cell body, or ellipsoid (E), and cross-striated rootlets (fibrils) radiate from it into the ellipsoid, which contains several elongated mitochondria (M). At least one filament of the cilium appears to act as a splint for the lamellar body. The lamellae of the outer segments are different in rods and cones. In rods, which function in scotopic vision, the lamella consists of a stack of membranous hollow discs which are separated from the outer plasma membrane. In cones, the continuity between the folded membranes of the lamella and the surrounding plasma membrane is retained. Cones are concentrated in the fovea and function in photopic (bright light-color) vision. (×20,700)

Figure 2. Electron micrograph of pigment layer of retina. The outermost layer of the retina consists of cuboidal epithelial cells with round nuclei (N). Large melanin granules (MG) are positioned in the cytoplasm, particularly on the surface adjacent to the outer segments of the rods and cones. The outer segments are surrounded by numerous microvilli (Mv) of the cuboidal cells. The outer surface rests upon a basal lamina (BL) separated from the capillaries (Ca) of the choroid by the elastic and collagen fibers of Bruch's membrane. Adjacent pigment cells are united by desmosomes and tight junctions. The cells are filled with smooth-surfaced endoplasmic reticulum (SER). (×9,800)

Figure 3. Electron micrograph of ganglion layer of retina. This is not a true ganglion but bears the name because the cells of this layer resemble neurons in ganglia. The neurons of the ganglion-cell layers are large pear-shaped cells with eccentric nuclei (N). Free ribosomes and mitochondria are distributed randomly in the cytoplasm. Dendrites (De) of this cell synapse with processes of the bipolar cells. A single axon (A) becomes part of the optic nerve. (×6,400)

Figure 4. Electron micrograph of bipolar cell cytoplasm. Cells of the inner nuclear layer are bipolar cells which synapse with rods and cones on one end and ganglion cells on the other. These are neurons which possess oval dense nuclei, mitochondria, and free ribosomes. A special arrangement of rough-surfaced endoplasmic reticulum (ER) is commonly found. The membranes are arranged in layers of tubules. Small vesicles are found both within and between the rough-surfaced tubules. The precise function of this tubular array is unknown. The same arrangement of rough-surfaced endoplasmic reticulum may occur in the cell body of rods and cones. (×17,400)

316

PLATE 143

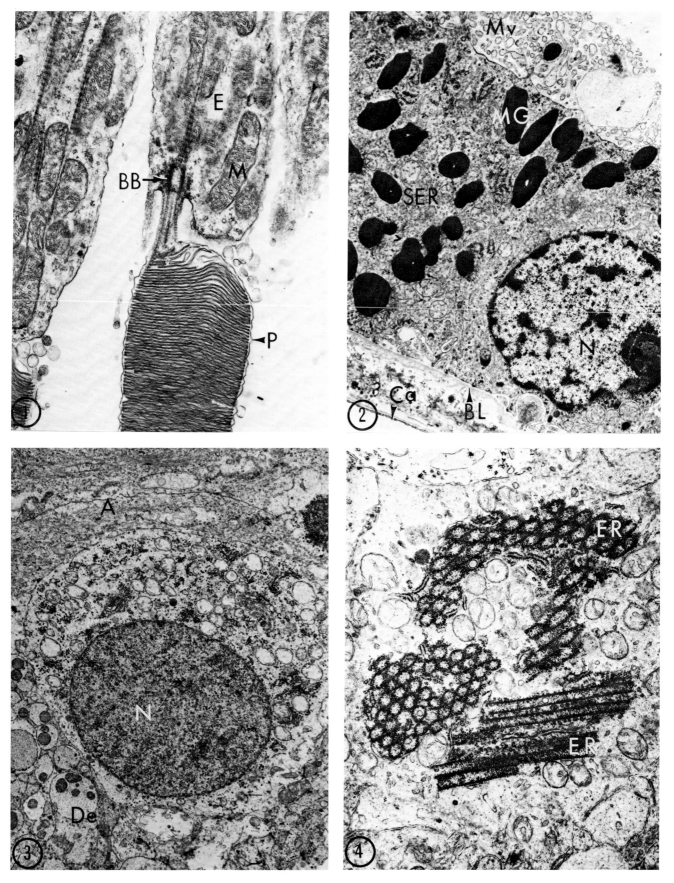

Plate 144 — INNER EAR

Figure 1.   Photomicrograph of cochlea. The bony labyrinth consists of a bony tube spiraling around a bony pillar, the modiolus (Mo). The basilar membrane (BM) bridges the osseous spiral lamina (OSL) and the spiral ligament (SL). The basilar membrane is the floor of the cochlear duct (CD), the roof of which is called Reissner's membrane (RM). Reissner's membrane is thin and consists of a double layer of squamous epithelial cells. The cochlear duct is situated between the scala vestibuli (SV) and the scala tympani (ST). The organ of Corti is a specialized group of cells lying on the floor of the cochlear duct. Connective tissue and tall columnar cells constitute the spiral limbus (SLi) bulging into the duct. Below this, axons of bipolar ganglion cells extend toward the cells of the organ of Corti. The outer margin of the limbus forms a groove, the internal spiral sulcus. Above this sulcus, the tectorial membrane (TM) extends from the lip of the limbus and contacts the hair cells of the organ of Corti supported by pillar and phalangeal cells. ($\times$60)

Figure 2.   Photomicrograph of organ of Corti. Cells of the organ of Corti rest upon the basal membrane (BL) which is lined on the side facing the scala tympani (ST) by squamous cells. Axons (A) of the bipolar cells occupy the connective tissue below the limbus (L). The lip of the limbus (LL) and the inner hair cells (H) and pillar cells (P) bound the internal spiral sulcus (ISS). Outer phalangeal cells (PC) lie adjacent to the pillar cells bounding the tunnel of Corti (TC). The bundles of microtubules (Mt) of the pillar cells extend from the basal membrane and terminate at the hair cell apex in a phalanx. ($\times$375)

Figure 3.   Electron micrograph of organ of Corti. The basal membrane (BL) serves as the floor of the cochlear duct (CD) and the roof of the scala tympani (ST). At the tunnel of Corti, bundles of microtubules are very prominent in the pillar cells (PC). These microtubules terminate on hemidesmosomes (HD) at the basal lamina. Pillar cells and phalangeal cells serve as a base for hair cells. Afferent nerves (Ne) synapse with the hair cells at their base. ($\times$11,500)

Figure 4.   (Insert) Photomicrograph of spiral limbus. The epithelial cells covering the spiral limbus are columnar. The vestibular membrane (VM) (Reissner's membrane) is continuous with this columnar epithelium but undergoes a rapid transition to simple squamous epithelium. Myelinated nerve (Ne) fibers from the bipolar cells occupy the floor of the limbus. ($\times$375)

PLATE 144

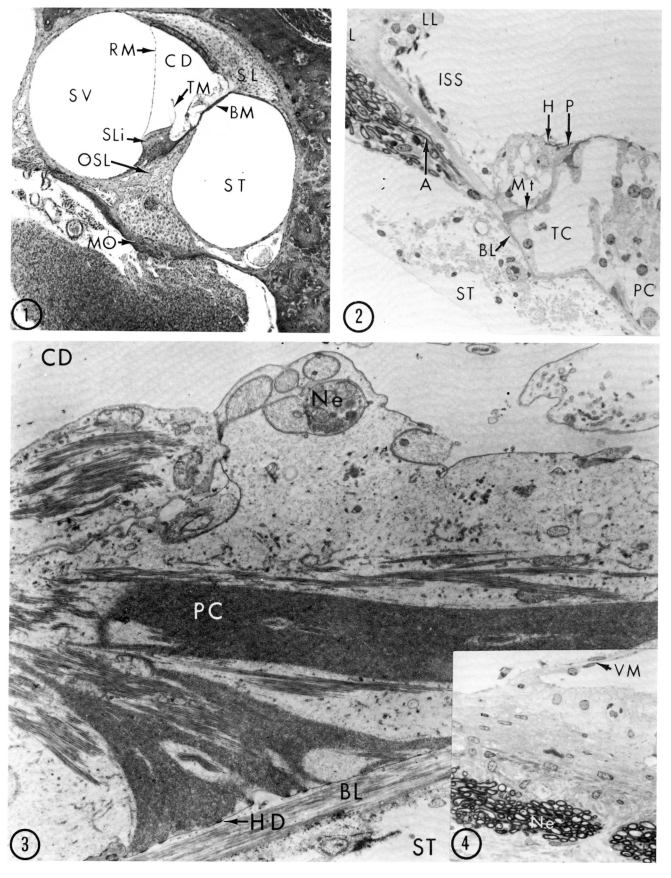

Plate 145 — INNER EAR: ORGAN OF CORTI

Figure 1. Electron micrograph of outer hair cells of organ of Corti. These outer hair cells (OHC) are elongated, with a centrally positioned nucleus (N). They become narrow at the apex and terminate in a conical-shaped cuticle which supports the auditory hairs; the cuticle is not seen in this view. The hair cells rest upon the body of subjacent outer phalangeal cells (Pg) originating at the basal lamina. Processes of the dendritic zone of the bipolar ganglion cells of the cochlear nerve (CN) travel to the hair cells and synapse on the base (Sn). The outer hair cells contain numerous small tubular-shaped mitochondria but other organelles are sparse. The phalangeal cells (Deiters' cells) contain smooth- and rough-surfaced endoplasmic reticulum and free ribosomes. Their mitochondria are large and spherical. ($\times$5,000)

Figure 2. Electron micrograph of inner hair cells and phalangeal cells of organ of Corti. The apical part of the hair cells (HC) contains a homogeneous dense fibrillar structure, the cuticle (Cu). The cuticle is cone shaped, with the base adjacent to the plasma membrane and the apex toward the cell interior. Cross sections of auditory hairs (AH) lie in the endolymphatic space. Mitochondria (M), rough-surfaced endoplasmic reticulum, free ribosomes, and small smooth-surfaced vesicles fill the cytoplasm. Hair cells are bounded laterally by phalangeal cells characterized by numerous microtubules (Mt) and united to the hair cells by tight junctions (TJ) and desmosomes (D). Bundles of microtubules extend from these junctional complexes at the apical border to the basilar lamina where they terminate in hemidesmosomes. ($\times$7,400)

Figure 3. Electron micrograph of efferent nerve at hair cell. The supportive phalangeal and pillar cells rest on the basal lamina and give support to the hair cells. These supportive cells extend a thin process called a phalanx (Ph) around the sides of the hair cells; this expands into a flat plate connected by junctional complexes (JC) to the hair cells (HC). The microtubules (Mt) originating at the base of these cells terminate upon the junctional complexes at the hair cells. The hair cells contain a homogeneous cuticle (Cu) in which a dense terminal web and basal bodies lie adjacent to the plasma membrane. Large mitochondria, smooth-surfaced vesicles and some lipid bodies occupy the peripheral cytoplasm. Rough-surfaced endoplasmic reticulum (ER) lines the lateral plasma membranes. The apex of the hair cells and the adjacent phalanx of the supportive cells together constitute the reticular lamina. Some large efferent nerve fibers (EN) are associated with hair cells. These axons synapse with the hair cells by short junctional complexes (JC). The axon contains mitochondria and an abundance of synaptic vesicles. ($\times$21,200)

Figure 4. Electron micrograph of hair cell. The bases of these cells rest in cup-like concavities of phalangeal cells. The apical cytoplasm contains mitochondria and membrane-limited vesicles having an osmophilic rim and a central void. These vesicles (V) are associated with the mitochondria. The cytoplasm bounding the lateral cell margins contains a single layer of rough-surfaced endoplasmic reticulum (ER). At the apex, a fibrillar cuticle contains terminal web fibers (TW) and basal bodies (BB). Cilial remnants extend from these basal bodies into the interior of the auditory hairs. The hairs (H) are microvilli narrow at their origin and flat and broadened at their free border. Microtubules (Mt) course from the basal bodies toward the cell base. The lateral margins of the hair cells are connected by junctional complexes (JC) to the flattened phalanges (Ph) of the adjacent phalangeal cells. ($\times$16,000)

320

PLATE 145

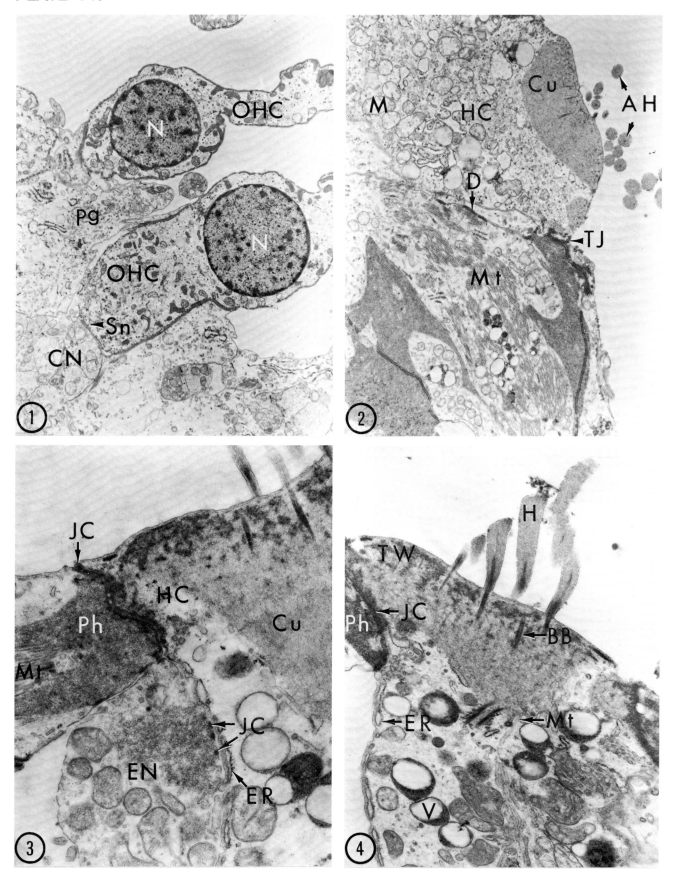

Integumentary System

PLATE 150

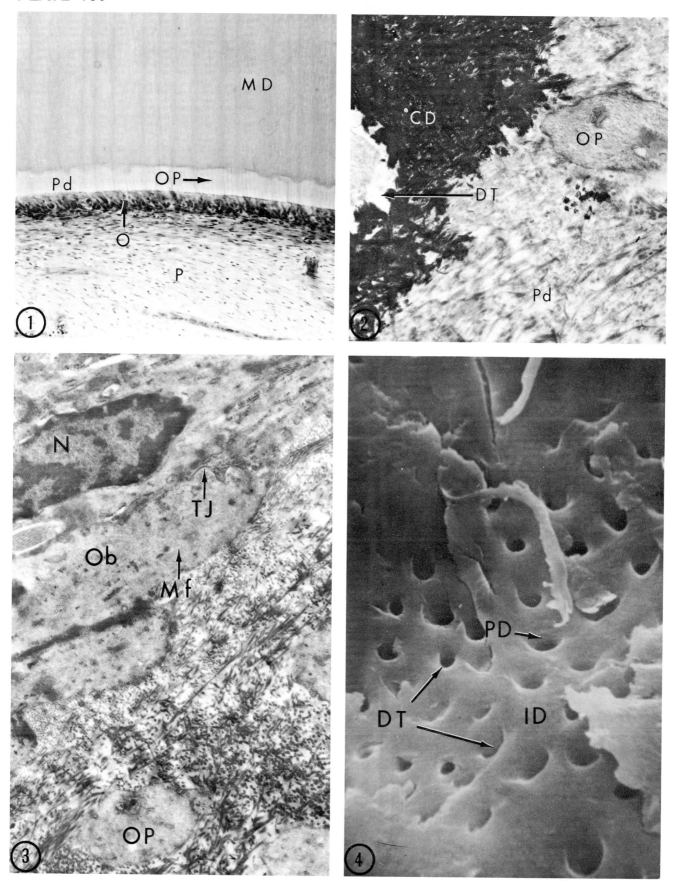

REFERENCES

The Cell

General References

Brachet, L.: *The Living Cell.* W. H. Freeman and Company, San Francisco, 1965.

Burke, J. D.: *Cell Biology.* Williams and Wilkins Company, Baltimore, 1970.

DeRobertis, E. N. and Saez, F. A.: *Cell Biology.* W. B. Saunders Company, Philadelphia, 1965.

Fawcett, D. W.: *An Atlas of Fine Structure. The Cell, Its Organelles and Inclusions.* W. B. Saunders Company, Philadelphia, 1966.

Laguens, R. P. and Dumm, C. L. A. G.: *Atlas of Human Electron Microscopy.* C. V. Mosby Company, St. Louis, 1969.

Porter, K. R. and Bonneville, M. A.: *An Introduction to the Fine Structure of Cells and Tissues,* ed. 3. Lea & Febiger, Philadelphia, 1968.

Rhodin, J. A. G.: *An Atlas of Ultrastructure.* W. B. Saunders Company, Philadelphia, 1963.

Sandborn, E. B.: *Cells and Tissues by Light and Electron Microscopy,* Vols. I and II. Academic Press, New York, 1970.

Warren, D. B. (ed.): *Formation and Fate of Cell Organelles,* Vol. 6. 1968.

Nucleus, Nucleolus, and Nuclear Pores

Anderson, E. and Beams, H. W.: Evidence from electron micrographs for the passage of material through pores of the nuclear membrane. *J. Biophys. Biochem. Cytol.* 2:434, 1956.

Barnes, B. G. and Davis, J. M.: The structure of nuclear pores in mammalian tissue. *J. Ultrastruct. Res.* 3:131, 1959.

Bennett, H. S.: Fine structure of cell nucleus, chromosomes, nucleoli and membrane. *Rev. Mod. Phys.* 31:297, 1959.

Bernhard, W. and Granboulan, N.: Electron microscopy of the nucleolus in vertebrate cells. In *Ultrastructure in Biological Systems* (Dalton, A. J. and Haguenau, F., eds.). Academic Press, New York, 1968.

Bertalanffy, F. D.: Tritiated thymidine vs. colchicine technique in the study of cell population cytodynamics. *Lab. Invest.* 13:871, 1964.

Feldherr, C. M.: The nuclear annuli as pathways for nucleocytoplasmic exchanges. *J. Cell Biol.* 14:65, 1962.

Gurdon, J. B.: Transplanted nuclei and cell differentiation. *Sci. Amer.* 219(6):24, 1968.

Maul, G. G.: Ultrastructure of pore complexes of annulate lamellae. *J. Cell Biol.* 46:604, 1970.

Miyai, K. and Steiner, J. W.: Fine structure of interphase liver cell nuclei in subacute ethionine intoxication. *Exp. Molec. Path.* 4:525, 1965.

Monneron, A. and Bernhard, W.: Fine structural organization of the interphase nucleus in some mammalian cells. *J. Ultrastruct. Res.* 27:266, 1969.

Porter, K. R.: Problems in the study of nuclear fine structure. In *Fourth International Conference of Electron Microscopy.* Springer-Verlag, Berlin, 1960.

Recher, L., Whitescarver, J. and Briggs, L.: A cytochemical and radioautographic study of human tissue culture cell nucleoli. *J. Cell Biol.* 45:479, 1970.

Wiener, J., Spiro, D. and Liewenstein, W. R.: Ultrastructure and permeability of nuclear membranes. *J. Cell Biol.* 27:107, 1965.

Chromosomes

Barnicott, N. A. and Huxley, H. E.: Electron microscope observations on mitotic chromosomes. *Quart. J. Micr. Sci. 106*:197, 1965.

Bergsma, D., Hamerton, J. L. and Klinger, H. P. (eds.): Birth defects. In *Chicago Conference: Standardization in Human Cytogenetics*. Original Article Series, Vol. 2, No. 2. The National Foundation, New York, 1966.

Crick, F. H. C.: The structure of the hereditary material. Reprinted from *Scientific American*, October, 1954.

Ford, E. H. R., Thurley, K. and Woollam, D. H. M.: Electron microscopic observations on whole human mitotic chromosomes. *J. Anat. 103*:143, 1968.

Gall, J. G.: On the submicroscopic structure of chromosomes. Mutation. *Brookhaven Sympos. Biol. 8*:17, 1956.

Moses, M. J.: The nucleus and chromosomes: A cytological perspective. In *Cytology and Cell Physiology* (Barne, G., ed.). Academic Press, New York, 1964.

Osgood, E. E., Jenkins, D. P., Brooks, R. and Lawson, R. K.: Electron micrographic studies of the expanded and uncoiled chromosomes from human leukocytes. *Ann. N. Y. Acad. Sci. 113*:717, 1963.

Priest, J. H.: *Cytogenetics.* Lea & Febiger, Philadelphia, 1969.

Priest, J. H. and Shikes, R. H.: Distribution of labeled chromatin. *J. Cell Biol. 47*:99, 1970.

Mitochondria

Harris, R. A., Williams, C. H., Caldwell, M. and Green, D. E.: Energized configurations of heart mitochondria in situ. *Science 165*:700, 1969.

Kurahasi, K., Tokunaga, J., Fujita, T. and Miyahara, M.: Scanning electron microscopy of isolated mitochondria I. *Arch. Histol. Jap. 30*:217, 1969.

Lehninger, A. L.: *The Mitochondrion-Molecular Basis of Structure and Function.* W. A. Benjamin, Inc., New York, 1964.

Mikulska, E., Odintsoua, M. S. and Turischeua, M. S.: Electron microscopy of DNA in mitochondria of pea seedlings. *J. Ultrastruct. Res. 32*:285, 1970.

Moran, H. F., Oda, T., Blair, P. V. and Green, D. E.: A macromolecular repeating unit of mitochondrial structure and function. *J. Cell Biol. 22*:63, 1964.

Muscatello, U. and Guarriero-Babyleua, V.: Effect of negative stains used in electron microscopy on some biochemical parameters of the mitochondrial activity. *J. Ultrastruct. Res. 31*:337, 1970.

Novikoff, A.: Mitochondria. In *The Cell* (Brachet, J. and Mirsky, A. E., eds.). Academic Press, New York, 1961.

Racker, E.: Resolution and reconstitution of the inner mitochondrial membrane. *Fed. Proc. 26*:1335, 1967.

Siekevitz, P.: Powerhouse of the cell. Reprinted from *Scientific American,* July, 1957.

Wills, E. J.: Crystalline structures in the mitochondria of normal human liver parenchymal cells. *J. Cell Biol. 24*:511, 1965.

Yamamoto, T.: On the relationship between mitochondria and fat droplets in the hepatic cells of the mouse after administration of hydrocortisone. *Arch. Histol. Jap. 15*:625, 1958.

Endoplasmic Reticulum and Ribosomes

Alfrey, V. G.: Nuclear ribosomes, messenger RNA and protein synthesis. *Exp. Cell Res. 9*(Suppl.):183, 1963.

338

Cotter, R. I., McPhie, P. and Gratzer, W. B.: Internal organization of the ribosome. *Nature 216*:864, 1967.

Haguenan, F.: The ergastoplasm: Its history, ultrastructure and biochemistry. *Int. Rev. Cytol. 7*:425, 1958.

Krishan, A.: Ribosome-granular material complexes in human leukemic lymphoblasts exposed to vinblastin sulfate. *J. Ultrastruct. Res. 31*:272, 1970.

Leblond, C. P. and Warren, K. B.: *The Use of Radioautography in Investigating Protein Synthesis.* Academic Press, New York, 1965.

Osawa, S.: Ribosome formation and structure. *Ann. Rev. Biochem. 37*:109, 1968.

Porter, K. R.: Observations on a submicroscopic basophilic component of the cytoplasm. *J. Exp. Med. 97*:727, 1953.

Rich, A.: Polyribosomes. *Sci. Amer. 209*:44, 1963.

Golgi Complex

Beams, H. W. and Kessel, R. G.: The Golgi apparatus: Structure and function. *Int. Rev. Cytol. 23*:209, 1968.

Caro, L.: Electron microscopic radioautography of thin sections. The Golgi zone as a site of protein concentration in pancreatic acinar cells. *J. Biophys. Biochem. Cytol. 10*:37, 1961.

Dalton, A. J.: Golgi apparatus and secretion granules. In *The Cell* (Brachet, J. and Mirsky, A. E., eds.). Academic Press, New York, 1961.

Glaumann, H. and Ericsson, J. L. E.: Evidence for the participation of the Golgi apparatus in the intracellular transport of nascent albumin in the liver cell. *J. Cell Biol. 47*:555, 1970.

Hicks, R. M.: The function of the Golgi complex in transitional epithelium. Synthesis of the thick cell membrane. *J. Cell Biol. 30*:623, 1966.

Maul, G. G.: On the relationship between the Golgi apparatus and annulate lamellae. *J. Ultrastruct. Res. 30*:368, 1970.

Mollenhauer, H. H., Moore, D. J. and Bergmann, L.: Homology of form in plant and animal Golgi apparatus. *Anat. Rec. 158*:313, 1967.

Palade, G. E.: The secretory process of the pancreatic exocrine cell. In *Electron Microscopy in Anatomy* (Boyd, J. D., Johnson, F. R. and Lever, J. D., eds.). Williams and Wilkins Company, Baltimore, 1961.

Palay, S. L.: The morphology of secretion. In *Frontiers in Cytology* (Palay, S. L., ed.). Yale University Press, New Haven, 1958.

Centrioles, Spindle Fibers and Cell Division

Ackerman, G. A.: Histochemistry of the centrioles and centrosomes of the leukemic cells from leukemic cells from human myeloblastic leukemia. *J. Biophys. Biochem. Cytol. 11*:717, 1961.

Allison, A. C.: Lysosomes. In *The Biological Basis of Medicine* (Bittar, E. E. and Bittar, N., eds.). Academic Press, New York, 1968.

Mazia, D.: How cells divide. *Sci. Amer. 105*(3):101, 1961.

O'Hara, P. T.: Spiral tilt of triplet fibers in human leukocyte centrioles. *J. Ultrastruct. Res. 31*:195, 1970.

Yamada, E.: Some observations on the fine structure of the centriole in the mitotic cell. *Kurume Med. J. 5*:36, 1958.

Lysosomes

DeDuve, C.: Lysosomes, a new group of cytoplasmic particles. In *Subcellular Particles* (Hayashi, T., ed.). Ronald Press, New York, 1958.

Dingle, J. T. and Fell, H. B. (eds.): *Lysosomes in Biology and Pathology*. John Wiley and Sons, New York, 1969.

Gahan, P. B.: Histochemistry of lysosomes. *Int. Rev. Cytol. 21*:1, 1967.

Helminen, H. J. and Ericsson, J. L.: On the mechanism of lysosomal enzyme secretion. Electron microscopic and histochemical studies on the epithelial cells of the rat's ventral prostate lobe. *J. Ultrastruct. Res. 33*:528, 1970.

Novikoff, A. B.: Lysosomes and related particles. In *The Cell* (Brachet, J. and Mirsky, A. E., eds.). Academic Press, New York, 1961.

Cell Inclusions, Glycogen, Lipids, Proteins, Pigments

Bennett, G.: Migration of glycoprotein from Golgi apparatus to cell coat in the columnar cells of the duodenal epithelium. *J. Cell Biol. 45*:668, 1970.

Biava, C.: Identification and structural forms of human particulate glycogen. *Lab. Invest. 12*:1179, 1963.

Bjoorkerud, S.: Isolation of lipofuscin granules from bovine cardiac muscle. *J. Ultrastruct. Res. 5*(Suppl.):5, 1963.

Drochmans, P.: Morphologie du glycogène. Étude au microscope electronique do colorations négatives du glycogène particulaire. *J. Ultrastruct. Res. 6*:141, 1962.

Duguid, J. B. and Lambert, M. W.: The pathogenesis of coal miners pneumoconiosis. *J. Path. Bact. 88*:389, 1964.

Essner, E. and Novikoff, A.: Human hepatocellular pigments and lysosomes. *J. Ultrastruct. Res. 3*:374, 1960.

Malkoff, D. and Strehler, B.: The ultrastructure of isolated and in situ human cardiac age pigment. *J. Cell Biol. 16*:611, 1963.

Revel, J. P.: Electron microscopy of glycogen. *J. Histochem. Cytochem. 12*:104, 1964.

Senior, J. R.: Intestinal absorption of fats. *J. Lipid Res. 5*:495, 1964.

Seiji, M., Birbeck, M. S. and Fitzpatrick, T. B.: Subcellular localization of melanin biosynthesis. *Ann. N. Y. Acad. Sci. 100*:497, 1963.

Themann, H.: Zur elektronenmikrosckopischen darstellung von glykogen mit Best's carmin. *J. Ultrastruct. Res. 4*:401, 1960.

Vye, M. V. and Fischman, D. A.: The morphological alteration of particulate glycogen by Enbloc staining with uranyl acetate. *J. Ultrastruct. Res. 33*:278, 1970.

Epithelium

Barber, V. C. and Boyde, A.: Scanning electron microscopic studies of cilia. *Z. Zellforsch. 84*:269, 1968.

Brody, I.: Variations in the differentiation of the fibrils in the normal human stratum corneum as revealed by electron microscopy. *J. Ultrastruct. Res. 30*:601, 1970.

Buschmann, R. J. and Taylor, A. B.: Extraction of absorbed lipid (linoleic acid-1-^{14}C) from rat intestinal epithelium during processing for electron microscopy. *J. Cell Biol. 38*:252, 1968.

Dunn, J. S.: The fine structure of the absorptive epithelial cells of the developing small intestine of the rat. *J. Anat. 101*:57, 1967.

Farquhar, M. G. and Palade, G. F.: Junctional complexes in various epithelia. *J. Cell Biol. 17*:375, 1963.

Frithiof, L.: Ultrastructural changes in the plasma membrane in human oral epithelium. *J. Ultrastruct. Res. 32*:1, 1970.

Hackemann, M., Grubb, C. and Hill, K. R.: The ultrastructure of normal squamous epithelium of the human cervix uteri. *J. Ultrastruct. Res. 22*:443, 1968.

Hayward, A. F.: An electron microscopic study of developing gall bladder and epithelium in the rabbit. *J. Anat. 100*:245, 1966.

Hayward, A. F.: The ultrastructure of developing gastric parietal cells in the foetal rabbit. *J. Anat. 101*:69, 1967.

Hicks, R. M.: The fine structure of the transitional epithelium of rat ureter. *J. Cell Biol. 26*:25, 1965.

Meader, R. D. and Landers, D. F.: Electron and light microscopic observations on relationships between lymphocytes and intestinal epithelium. *Amer. J. Anat. 121*:763, 1967.

Mukherjee, T. M. and Williams, A. W.: A comparative study of the ultrastructure of microvilli in the epithelium of small and large intestine of mice. *J. Cell Biol. 34*:447, 1967.

Satir, P.: Cilia. *Sci. Amer. 204*:61, 1961.

Sorokin, S. P.: Reconstruction of centriole formation and ciliogenesis in mammalian lungs. *J. Cell Sci. 3*:207, 1968.

Susi, F. R., Belt, W. D. and Kelly, J. W.: Fine structure of fibrillar complexes associated with the basement membrane in human oral mucosa. *J. Cell Biol. 34*:686, 1967.

Zelickson, A. S.: *Ultrastructure of Normal and Abnormal Skin.* Lea & Febiger, Philadelphia, 1967.

Connective and Supporting Tissue

Fibers

Carmichael, C. G. and Fullmer, H. M.: The fine structure of the oxytalan fiber. *J. Cell Biol. 28*:33, 1966.

Chapman, J. A., Kellgren, J. H. and Steven, F. S.: Assembly of collagen fibrils. *Fed. Proc. 25*:1811, 1966.

Fahrenback, W. H., Sandberg, L. B. and Cleary, E. G.: Ultrastructural studies on early elastogenesis. *Anat. Rec. 155*:563, 1966.

Gould, B. S. (ed.): *Treatise on Collagen. Biology of Collagen*, Vol. 2, Parts A and B. Academic Press, New York, 1968.

Grant, R. A., Cox, R. W. and Horne, R. W.: The structure and assembly of collagen fibrils. 2. An electron-microscope study of cross-linked collagen. *J. Roy. Micr. Soc. 87*:143, 1967.

Greenlee, T. K., Jr., Ross, R. and Palade, G. E.: The fine structure of elastic fibers. *J. Cell Biol. 30*:59, 1966.

Higgs, D. G. and Reed, R.: Electron microscope studies of reconstituted eucollagen. *Biochim. Biophys. Acta 78*:265, 1963.

McGavin, S. and Pyper, A. S.: An electron-microscope study of elastoidin. *Biochim. Biophys. Acta 79*:600, 1964.

Myers, D. B., Highton, T. C. and Rayns, D. G.: Acid mucopolysaccharides closely associated with collagen fibrils in normal human synovium. *J. Ultrastruct. Res.* 28:203, 1969.

Revel, J. P. and Hay, E. D.: An autoradiographic and electron microscopic study of collagen synthesis in differentiating cartilage. *Z. Zellforsch.* 61:110, 1963.

Rhodin, J. A. G.: Organization and ultrastructure of connective tissue. In *The Connective Tissue* (Wagner, B. M. and Smith, D. E., eds.). Williams and Wilkins Company, Baltimore, 1967.

Ross, R.: Wound healing and collagen formation. V. Quantitative electron microscope radioautographic observations of proline in H3 utilization by fibroblasts. *J. Cell Biol.* 27:83, 1965.

Taylor, J. J. and Yeager, J. L.: The fine structure of elastic fibers in the fibrous periosteum of the rat femur. *Anat. Rec.* 156:129, 1966.

Ground Substance

DuPraw, E. J.: Physical chemistry of macromolecules. In *Cell and Molecular Biology.* Academic Press, New York, 1968.

Hall, D. A. (ed.): *International Review of Connective Tissue Research,* Vols. 1, 2, and 3. Academic Press, New York, 1963, 1964, 1965.

Johansson, B. I., Persson, I. and Manera, P.: Histologic effects of collagen and chondroitin sulphate as capping agents in amputated rat molar pulps. *Arch. Oral Biol.* 8:503, 1963.

Olsen, B. R.: Electron microscopy studies on collagen. IV. Structure of vitrosin fibrils and interaction properties of vitrosin molecules. *J. Ultrastruct. Res.* 13:172, 1965.

Olsen, B. R.: Electron microscopy studies on collagen. V. The structure of segment-long-spacing aggregates consisting of molecules renatured from the isolated fraction of rat tail tendon collagen. *J. Ultrastruct. Res.* 19:432, 1967.

Olsen, B. R.: Electron microscopy studies on collagen. VI. The structure of segment-long-spacing aggregates consisting of molecules renatured from isolated fractions of codfish skin collagen. *J. Ultrastruct. Res.* 19:446, 1967.

General Connective Tissue Cells—Areolar Tissue

Bois, P.: Mast cells and histamine concentration in muscle and liver of dystrophic mice. *Amer. J. Physiol.* 206:338, 1964.

Braunsteiner, H., Fellinger, K. and Pakesch, F.: Demonstration of a cytoplasmic structure in plasma cells. *Blood* 8:916, 1953.

Brewer, D. B.: Electron-microscope observations on the phagocytosis of neutrophil polymorphonuclear leucocytes by macrophages. *J. Path. Bact.* 88:307, 1964.

Chapman, J. A., Gough, J. and Elves, M. W.: An electron microscopic study of the *in vitro* transformation of human leucocytes. II. Transformation to macrophages. *J. Cell Sci.* 2:371, 1967.

Coons, A. H., Leduc, E. H. and Connolly, J. M.: Studies on antibody production. I. A method for the histochemical demonstration of specific antibody and its application to a study of the hyper-immune rabbit. *J. Exp. Med.* 102:49, 1955.

dePetris, S., Karlsbad, G. and Pernis, B.: Localization of antibodies in plasma cells by electron microscopy. *J. Exp. Med.* 117:849, 1963.

Fujita, H., Asagami, C., Murozimu, S., Yamamoto, K. and Kinoshita, K.: Electron microscopic studies of mast cells of human fetal skins. *J. Ultrastruct. Res.* 28:353, 1969.

Greenlee, T. K.: The fine structure changes in differentiation of tendon fibroblasts. *Southern Med. J. 61:*711, 1968.

Harris, W. H. and Heaney, R. P.: *Skeletal Renewal and Metabolic Bone Disease.* Little, Brown and Company, Boston, 1969.

Hori, W., Toda, K., Pathak, M. S., Clark, W. H. and Fitzpatrick, T. B.: A fine-structure study of the human epidermal melanosome complex and its acid phosphatase activity. *J. Ultrastruct. Res. 25:*109, 1968.

Hummeler, K., Harris, S. and Harris, T. N.: Fine structure of some antibody-producing cells. *Fed. Proc. 25:*1734, 1966.

Jackson, S. F.: Connective tissue cells. In *The Cell* (Brachet, J. and Mirsky, A. E., eds.). Academic Press, New York, 1964.

Kajikawa, K.: Electron microscopic studies on histiocytes. *Tohoku J. Exp. Med. 81:*350, 1964.

Kobayashi, T., Midtgard, K. and Asboe-Hansen, G.: Ultrastructure of human mast-cell granules. *J. Ultrastruct. Res. 23:*153, 1968.

Lindell, T. J., Weinberg, F., Morris, P. W., Roeder, R. G. and Rutter, W. J.: Macrophage membranes viewed through a scanning electron microscope. *Science 170:*446, 1970.

Movat, H. A. and Fernando, N. V. P.: The fine structure of connective tissue. II. The plasma cells. *Exp. Molec. Path. 1:*535, 1962.

Napolitano, L.: The differentiation of white adipose cells. An electron microscope study. *J. Cell Biol. 18:*663, 1963.

Padawer, J.: Microtubules in rat peritoneal fluid mast cells. *J. Cell Biol. 35:*180A, 1967.

Rifkind, R. A., Osserman, E. F., Hsu, K. C. and Morgan, C.: The intracellular distribution of gamma globulin in a mouse plasma cell tumor as revealed by fluorescence and electron microscopy. *J. Exp. Med. 116:*423, 1962.

Ross, R.: The connective tissue fiber forming cell. In *Treatise on Collagen* (Gould, B. S., ed.). Academic Press, New York, 1968.

Sagebiel, R. W. and Reed, T. H.: Serial reconstruction of the characteristic granule of the Langerhans cell. *J. Cell Biol. 36:*595, 1968.

Sainte-Marie, G.: Study on plasmacytopoiesis. I. Mediastinal lymph nodes of ten week old rats. *Amer. J. Anat. 114:*207, 1964.

Selye, H.: *The Mast Cell.* Butterworth, London and Washington, 1965.

Storb, U. and Weiser, R. S.: Antibody-carrying cells in the immune response. 1. Identification of "rosette" forming cells by light microscopy. *J. Reticuloendothel. Soc. 4:*51, 1967.

Szakacs, A., Sinkovics, J. G., Butler, J. J. and Levy, B. M.: Electron microscopic observations of the interaction of macrophages and lymphocytes in a virus-induced murine lymphoma. *J. Infect. Dis. 118:*240, 1968.

Taichman, N. S.: Ultrastructure of guinea pig mast cells. *J. Ultrastruct. Res. 32:*284, 1970.

Weinstock, A.: Plasma cells in human gingiva: An electron microscopic study. *Anat. Rec. 162:*289, 1968.

Zelickson, A. S.: Fibroblast development and fibrogenesis. A histochemical and electron microscope study. *Arch. Derm. 88:*497, 1963.

Cartilage

Kuettner, K. E., Sobel, L. W., Ray, R. D., Croxen, R. L., Passovoy, M. and Eisenstein, R.: Lysozyme in epiphyseal cartilage. *J. Cell Biol. 44:*329, 1970.

Matthews, J. L., Martin, J. H. and Collins, E. J.: Metabolism of radioactive calcium by cartilage. *Clin. Orthop. 58:*213, 1968.

Matthews, J. L., Martin, J. H., Lynn, J. A. and Collins, E. J.: Calcium incorporation in the developing cartilaginous epiphysis. *Calc. Tiss. Res. 1:*330, 1968.

Palfrey, A. J. and Davies, D. V.: The fine structure of chondrocytes. *J. Anat. 100:*213, 1966.

Roy, S.: Ultrastructure of articular cartilage in experimental hemarthrosis. *Arch. Path. 86:*69, 1968.

Ruttner, J. R. and Spycher, M. A.: Electron microscopic investigations on aging and osteoarthritic human cartilage. *Path. Microbiol. 31:*14, 1968.

Schenk, R. K., Spiro, D. and Wiener, J.: Cartilage resorption in the tibial epiphyseal plate of growing rats. *J. Cell Biol. 34:*275, 1967.

Schenk, R. K., Wiener, J. and Spiro, D.: Fine structural aspects of vascular invasion of the tibial epiphyseal plate of growing rats. *Acta Anat. 69:*1, 1968.

Silberberg, M., Silberberg, R. and Hasler, M.: Fine structure of articular cartilage in mice receiving cortisone acetate. *Arch. Path. 82:*569, 1966.

Silberberg, M., Silberberg, R. and Hasler, M.: Early effects of somatotrophin on the fine structure of articular cartilage. *Anat. Rec. 151:*297, 1965.

Bone

Ascenzi, A., Bonucci, E. and Bocciarelli, D. S.: An electron microscope study on primary periosteal bone. *J. Ultrastruct. Res. 18:*605, 1967.

Baud, C. A.: Submicroscopic structure and functional aspects of the osteocyte. *Clin. Orthop. 56:*227, 1968.

Blanden, R. V.: Modification of macrophage function. *J. Reticuloendothel. Soc. 5:*179, 1968.

Boyde, A. and Hobdell, M. H.: Scanning electron microscopy of primary membrane bone. *Z. Zellforsch. 99:*98, 1969.

Cameron, D. A., Paschall, H. A. and Robinson, R. A.: Changes in the fine structure of bone cells after the administration of parathyroid extract. *J. Cell Biol. 33:*1, 1967.

Cooper, R. R., Milgram, J. W. and Robinson, R. A.: Morphology of the osteon: An electron microscopic study. *J. Bone Joint Surg. 48A:*1239, 1966.

Glimcher, M. J. and Krane, S. M.: The organization and structure of bone, and the mechanism of calcification. In *Treatise on Collagen* (Gould, B. S., ed.). Academic Press, New York, 1968.

Hobdell, M. H. and Boyde, A.: Microradiography and scanning electron microscopy of bone sections. *Z. Zellforsch. 94:*487, 1969.

Jones, S. J. and Boyde, A.: Experimental studies on the interpretation of bone surfaces studied with the scanning electron microscope. Scanning electron microscopy/1970. *Proceedings of the Third Annual Scanning Electron Microscopy Symposium.* Illinois Research Institute, Chicago, 1970.

Martin, J. H. and Matthews, J. L.: Mitochondrial granules in chondrocytes. *Calc. Tiss. Res. 3:*184, 1969.

Martin, J. H. and Matthews, J. L.: Mitochondrial granules in chondrocytes, osteoblasts and osteocytes. *Clin. Orthop. 68:*273, 1970.

Matthews, J. L., Martin, J. H., Race, G. J. and Collins, E. J.: Giant cell centrioles. *Science 155:*1423, 1967.

Matthews, J. L., Martin, J. H., Sampson, H. W., Kunin, A. S. and Roan, J. H.: Mitochondrial granules in the normal and rachitic rat epiphysis. *Calc. Tiss. Res. 5:91,* 1970.

Molnar, Z.: Additional observations on bone crystal dimensions. *Clin. Orthop. 17:38,* 1960.

Posner, A. S.: Relationship between diet and bone mineral ultrastructure. *Fed. Proc. 26:1717,* 1967.

Robinson, R. A. and Cameron, D. A.: Bone. In *Electron Microscopic Anatomy* (Kurtz, S. M., ed.). Academic Press, New York, 1964.

Rosse, C. and Clawson, D. K.: *Introduction to the Musculoskeletal System.* Harper and Row, New York, in press.

Woods, J. F. and Nichols, G., Jr.: Collagenolytic activity in rat bone cells. Characteristics and intracellular location. *J. Cell Biol. 26:747,* 1965.

Blood and Hemopoeises

Erythrocytes

Baker, R. F.: Ultrastructure of the red blood cell. *Fed. Proc. 26:1785,* 1967.

Blanton, P. L., Martin, J. H. and Haberman, S.: Pinocytotic response of circulating erythrocytes to specific blood grouping antibodies. *J. Cell Biol. 37:716,* 1968.

Campbell, F. R.: Nuclear elimination from the normoblast of fetal guinea pig liver as studied with electron microscopy and serial sectioning techniques. *Anat. Rec. 160:539,* 1968.

Harris, J. R. and Agutter, P.: A negative staining study of human erythrocyte ghosts and rat liver nuclear membranes. *J. Ultrastruct. Res. 33:219,* 1970.

Koehler, J. K.: Freeze-etching observations on nucleated erythrocytes with special reference to the nuclear and plasma membranes. *Z. Zellforsch. 85:1,* 1968.

Miller, D. M. and Hannay, C. L.: The electron microscopy of vesicles formed during the mechanical disruption of human erythrocytes. *Canad. J. Physiol. Pharmacol. 43:675,* 1965.

Skutelsky, E. and Danon, D.: An electron microscopic study of nuclear elimination from the late erythroblast. *J. Cell Biol. 33:625,* 1967.

Steward, G. J. and Turner, H. M.: Ultrastructural characteristics and behavior of previously frozen glycerolyzed, and deglycerolyzed human red blood cells. *Cryobiology 4:189,* 1968.

Granulocytes

Ackerman, G. A.: Ultrastructure and cytochemistry of the developing neutrophil. *Lab. Invest. 19:290,* 1968.

Anderson, D. R.: Ultrastructure of normal and leukemic leukocytes in human peripheral blood. *J. Ultrastruct. Res. 9*(Suppl.):1, 1966.

Bainton, D. F. and Farquhar, M. G.: Difference in enzyme content of azurophil and specific granules of polymorphonuclear leukocytes. II. Cytochemistry and electron microscopy of bone marrow cells. *J. Cell Biol. 39:299,* 1968.

Cooper, E. H. and Inman, D. R.: Ultrastructure of human leukocytes synthesizing DNA. *Nature 204:894,* 1964.

Dolowy, W. C., Cornet, J. and Henson, D.: Particles in leukocytes of normal human beings after negative staining in electron microscopy. *Nature 209:1358,* 1966.

Fedorko, M.: Effect of chloroquine on morphology of cytoplasmic granules in maturing human leukocytes. An ultrastructural study. *J. Clin. Invest. 46:*1932, 1967.

Fedorko, M.: Formation of cytoplasmic granules in human eosinophilic myelocytes: An electron microscopic autoradiographic study. *Blood 31:*188, 1968.

Franklin, D. A.: Electron microscopic study of human basophils. *Blood 29:*878, 1967.

Gerber, P. and Monroe, J. H.: Studies on leukocytes growing in continuous culture derived from normal human donors. *J. Nat. Cancer Inst. 40:*855, 1968.

Ghidoni, J. J. and Goldberg, A. F.: Light and electron microscope localization of acid phosphatase activity in human eosinophils. *Amer. J. Clin. Path. 45:*402, 1966.

Kaihotsu, N.: Electron microscopic studies on the maturation process of neutrophilic leucocytes. *Kobe J. Med. Sci. 13:*47, 1967.

Lockwood, W. R. and Allison, F., Jr.: Electron microscopy of phagocytic cells. 3. Morphological findings related to adhesive properties of human and rabbit granulocytes. *Brit. J. Exp. Path. 47:*158, 1966.

Lockwood, W. R. and Allison, F.: Electron micrographic studies of phagocytic cells. II. Observations on the changes induced in the cytoplasmic contents of human granulocytes by the ingestion of rough pneumococcus. *Brit. J. Exp. Path. 45:*294, 1964.

McDuffie, N. G.: Crystalline patterns in Auer bodies and specific granules of human leukocytes. *J. Microscopie 6:*321, 1967.

Miller, F., De Harven, E. and Palade, G. E.: The structure of eosinophil leukocyte granules in rodents and in man. *J. Cell Biol. 31:*349, 1966.

Ross, R. and Klebanoff, S. J.: The eosinophilic leukocyte. Fine structure studies of changes in the uterus during the estrous cycle. *J. Exp. Med. 124:*653, 1966.

Scott, R. E. and Horn, R. G.: Fine structural features of eosinophil granulocyte development in human bone marrow. *J. Ultrastruct. Res. 33:*16, 1970.

Wetzel, B. K., Horn, R. G. and Spicer, S. S.: Fine structure studies on the development of heterophil, eosinophil and basophil granulocytes in rabbits. *Lab. Invest. 16:*349, 1967.

Yamada, E.: Electron microscopy of the peroxidase in the granular leukocytes of rat bone marrow. *Arch. Histol. Jap. 27:*131, 1966.

Zucker-Franklin, D.: Electron microscopic study of human basophils. *Blood 29:*878, 1967.

Zucker-Franklin, D.: Electron microscopic studies of human granulocytes: Structural variations related to function. *Seminars Hemat. 5:*109, 1968.

Agranulocytes
Douglas, S. D., Hoffman, P. F., Borgeson, J. and Chessin, L. H.: Studies on human peripheral blood lymphocytes *in vitro.* Fine structural features of lymphocyte transformation by pokeweed antigen. *J. Immun. 98:*17, 1967.

Hann, S. S. and Johnson, A. G.: Radioautographic and electron-microscope evidence of rapid uptake of antigen by lymphocytes. *Science 153:*176, 1966.

Hovig, T., Jeremic, M. and Stavem, P.: A new type of inclusion bodies in lymphocytes. *Scand. J. Haemat. 5:*81, 1968.

Jamuar, M. P., Kim, C. W. and Hamilton, L. D.: Fine structure of lymphocytes sensitized to Trichinella spiralis antigen. *J. Immun. 100:*329, 1968.

Johnson, F. R. and Roberts, D. B.: The growth and division of human small lymphocytes in tissue culture: An electron microscopic study. *J. Anat. 98:*303, 1964.

Lazarus, S. S., Vethamany, V. G. and Volk, B. W.: Fine structure of phytohemagglutinin transformed lymphocytes. *Arch. Path. 86*:176, 1968.

McFarland, W.: Microspikes on the lymphocyte uropod. *Science 163*:818, 1969.

Mollo, F., Stramignoni, A. and Volante, G.: Ricerche sui mononucleati del sangue umano in coltura. 2. Ultrastruttura delle cellule coltivate con fitoemagglutinina. *Pathologica 58*:23, 1966.

Sutton, J. S.: Ultrastructural aspects of *in vitro* development of monocytes into macrophages, epitheloid cells, and multinucleated giant cells. *Nat. Cancer Inst. Monog. 26*:71, 1967.

Sutton, J. S. and Weiss, L.: Transformation of monocytes in tissue culture into macrophages, epitheloid cells, and multinucleated giant cells. An electron microscope study. *J. Cell Biol. 28*:303, 1966.

Tokuyasu, K., Madden, S. C. and Zeldis, L. J.: Fine structural alterations of interphase nuclei of lymphocytes stimulated to growth activity *in vitro*. *J. Cell Biol. 39*:630, 1968.

Trowell, O. A.: Ultrastructural changes in lymphocytes exposed to noxious agents *in vitro*. *Quart. J. Exp. Physiol. 51*:207, 1966.

Weiss, L. and Aisenberg, A. C.: An electron microscope study of lymphatic tissue in runt disease. *J. Cell Biol. 25*:149, 1965.

Platelets

Behnke, O.: Electron microscopic observations on the membrane systems of the rat blood platelet. *Anat. Rec. 158*:121, 1967.

Behnke, O. and Zelander, T.: Filamentous substructure of microtubules of the marginal bundle of mammalian blood platelets. *J. Ultrastruct. Res. 19*:147, 1967.

Behnke, O.: Electron microscopical observations on the surface coating of human blood platelets. *J. Ultrastruct. Res. 24*:51, 1968.

Davis, R. B. and Kay, D.: Demonstration of 5-hydroxytryptamine in blood platelets by electron microscope autoradiography. *Nature 207*:650, 1965.

Johnson, S. A., Monto, R. W., Rebuck, J. W. and Horn, R. C. (eds.): *Blood Platelets*. Henry Ford Hospital International Symposium. Little, Brown and Company, Boston, 1960.

Johnson, S. A., Van Horn, D. L., Pederson, H. J. and Marr, J.: The function of platelets: A review. *Transfusion 6*:3, 1966.

Mustard, J. F., Glynn, M. F., Nishizawa, E. E. and Packham, M. A.: Platelet-surface interactions: Relationship to thrombosis and hemostases. *Fed. Proc. 26*:97, 1967.

Rodman, N. F. and Mason, R. G.: Platelet-platelet interaction: Relationship to hemostasis and thrombosis. *Fed. Proc. 26*:95, 1967.

White, J. G. and Krivit, W.: Fine structural localization of adenosine triphosphatase in human platelets and other blood cells. *Blood 26*:554, 1965.

Zucker-Franklin, D.: The submembranous fibrils of human blood platelets. *J. Cell Biol. 47*:293, 1970.

Zucker-Franklin, D., Nachman, R. L. and Marcus, A. J.: Ultrastructure of thrombosthenin, the contractile protein of human blood platelets. *Science 157*:945, 1967.

Marrow

Behnke, O.: An electron microscope study of the megakaryocyte of the rat bone marrow. 1. The development of the demarcation membrane system and the platelet surface coat. *J. Ultrastruct. Res. 24*:412, 1968.

Bessis, M.: The blood cells and their formation. In *The Cell* (Brachet, J. and Mirsky, A. E., eds.). Academic Press, New York, 1961.

Capone, R. J., Weinreb, E. L. and Chapman, G. B.: Electron microscope studies on normal human myeloid elements. *Blood 23*:300, 1964.

Goodman, J. R., Wallerstein, R. A. and Hall, S. G.: The ultrastructure of bone marrow histiocytes in megaloblastic anaemia and the anaemia of infection. *Brit. J. Haemat. 14*:471, 1968.

Hudson, G.: Eosinophil granules and uranyl acetate. An electron microscopic study of guinea-pig bone marrow. *Exp. Cell Res. 46*:121, 1967.

Hudson, G.: Eosinophil granules and cell maturity: Electron microscopic observations on guinea-pig marrow. *Acta Haemat. 36*:350, 1966.

Hudson, G.: Eosinophil granules and phosphotungstic acid: An electron microscopic study of guinea-pig bone marrow. *Exp. Cell Res. 41*:265, 1966.

Scott, R. E. and Horn, R. G.: Fine structural features of eosinophil granulocyte development in human bone marrow. *J. Ultrastruct. Res. 33*:16, 1970.

Wetzel, B. K., Horn, R. G. and Spicer, S. S.: Fine structure studies of the development of heterophil, eosinophil, and basophil granulocytes in rabbits. *Lab. Invest. 16*:349, 1967.

Lymphoid Organs

Bartman, J., Van de Veide, R. L. and Friedman, F.: Pigmented lipid histiocytosis and susceptibility to infection: Ultrastructure of splenic histiocytes. *Pediatrics 40*:1000, 1967.

Chan, G., Rancourt, M. W., Ceglowski, W. S. and Friedman, H.: Leukemia virus suppression of antibody-forming cells: Ultrastructure of infected spleens. *Science 159*:437, 1968.

Edwards, V. D. and Simon, G. T.: Ultrastructural aspects of red cell destruction in the normal rat spleen. *J. Ultrastruct. Res. 33*:187, 1970.

Mollo, G. and Stramignoni, A.: Cytoplasmic fibrillar ultrastructures in human lymph node cells. *Estratto da Atti del V Congresso Italiano di Microscopia Elettronica.* Bologna, Ottobre, 1965.

Nossal, G. J., Abbot, A., Mitchell, J. and Lummus, Z.: Antigens in immunity. XV. Ultrastructural features of antigen capture in primary and secondary lymphoid follicles. *J. Exp. Med. 127*:277, 1968.

Yamada, E.: The fine structure of the megakaryocyte in the mouse spleen. *Acta Anat. 29*:267, 1957.

Muscle

Skeletal Muscle

Carlsen, F., Fuchs, F. and Knappeis, G. G.: Contractility and ultrastructure in glycerol-extracted muscle fibers. I. The relationship of contractility to sarcomere length. *J. Cell Biol. 27*:25, 1965.

Carlsen, F., Fuchs, F. and Knappeis, G. G.: Contractility and ultrastructure in glycerol-extracted muscle fibers. II. Ultrastructure in resting and shortened fibers. *J. Cell Biol. 27*:35, 1965.

Cheng-Minoda, K., Davidowitz, J., Liebowitz, A. and Breinin, G. M.: Fine structure of extraocular muscle in rabbit. *J. Cell Biol. 39*:193, 1968.

Cornog, J. L. and Gonatas, N. K.: Ultrastructure of rhabdomyoma. *J. Ultrastruct. Res.* *20*:433, 1967.

Engel, A. G.: Ultrastructural reactions in muscle disease. *Med. Clin. N. Amer.* *52*:909, 1968.

Engel, A. G. and Dale, A. J.: Autophagic glycogenosis of late onset with mitochondrial abnormalities: Light and electron microscopic observations. *Mayo Clin. Proc.* *43*:233, 1968.

Goldfischer, S.: The cytochemical localization of myoglobin in striated muscle of man and walrus. *J. Cell Biol.* *34*:398, 1967.

Gonatas, N. K., Perez, M. C., Shy, G. M. and Evangelista, I.: Central "core" disease of skeletal muscle. Ultrastructural and cytochemical observations in two cases. *Amer. J. Path.* *47*:503, 1965.

Huxley, H. E.: The contraction of muscle. *Sci. Amer.* *199*(4):67, 1958.

Ikemoto, N., Kitagawa, S., Nakamura, A. and Gergely, J.: Electron microscopic investigations of actomyosin as a function of ionic strength. *J. Cell Biol.* *39*:620, 1968.

Jones, J. K., Cohen, C., Szent-Gyorgyi, A. G. and Longley, W.: Paramyosin: Molecular length and assembly. *Science* *163*:1196, 1969.

Knappeis, G. G. and Carlsen, F.: The ultrastructure of the M line in skeletal muscle. *J. Cell Biol.* *38*:202, 1968.

McCallister, L. P. and Hadek, R.: Transmission electron microscopy and stereo ultrastructure of the T system in frog skeletal muscle. *J. Ultrastruct. Res.* *33*:203, 1970.

Mintz, G., Gonzalez-Angulo, A., Fraga, A. and Zavala, B. J.: Ultrastructure of muscle in polymyositis. *Amer. J. Med.* *44*:216, 1968.

Pepe, F. A.: The myosin filament. 1. Structural organization from antibody staining observed in electron microscopy. *J. Molec. Biol.* *27*:203, 1967.

Reger, J. F. and Craig, A. S.: Studies on the fine structure of muscle fibers and associated satellite cells in hypertrophic human deltoid muscle. *Anat. Rec.* *162*:483, 1968.

Resnick, J. S., Engel, W. K. and Nelson, P. G.: Changes in the Z disk of skeletal muscle induced by tenotomy. *Neurology* *18*:737, 1968.

Samaha, F. J.: Human striated muscle myofibrils and actomyosin. *Neurology* *17*:1152, 1967.

Shafia, S. A., Gorycki, M., Goldstone, L. and Milhorat, A. T.: The fine structure of fiber types in normal human muscle. *Anat. Rec.* *156*:283, 1966.

Walker, S. M., Schrodt, G. R. and Bingham, M.: Electron microscope study of sarcoplasmic reticulum at the Z line level in skeletal muscle fibers of fetal and newborn rats. *J. Cell Biol.* *39*:469, 1968.

Cardiac Muscle

Johnson, E. A. and Sommer, J. R.: A strand of cardiac muscle. Its ultrastructure and the electrophysiological implication of its geometry. *J. Cell Biol.* *33*:103, 1967.

Karnovsky, M. J.: The localization of cholinesterase activity in rat cardiac muscle by electron microscopy. *J. Cell Biol.* *23*:217, 1964.

Leak, L. V. and Burke, J. F.: The ultrastructure of human embryonic myocardium. *Anat. Rec.* *149*:623, 1964.

Legato, M. J., Spiro, D. and Langer, G. A.: Ultrastructural alterations produced in mammalian myocardium by variation in perfusate ionic compositions. *J. Cell Biol.* *37*:1, 1968.

McCallister, B. D. and Brown, A. L.: A quantitative study of myocardial mitochondria in experimental cardiac hypertrophy. *Lab. Invest.* 14:692, 1965.

Mizumo, S., Araya, K. and Takahashi, A.: An electron microscopic study of the myofilament of the mammalian cardiac muscular tissue. *Jap. Circ. J.* 29:1261, 1965.

Novi, A. M.: An electron microscopic study of the innervation of papillary muscles in the rat. *Anat. Rec.* 160:123, 1968.

Reichenback, D. D. and Benditt, E. P.: Myofibrillar degeneration. A response of the myocardial cell to injury. *Arch. Path.* 85:189, 1968.

Simpson, F. O.: The transverse tubular system in mammalian myocardial cells. *Amer. J. Anat.* 117:1, 1965.

Sjostrand, F. S. and Andersson-Cedergren, E.: Intercalated discs of heart muscle. In *The Structure and Function of Muscle* (Bourne, G., ed.). Academic Press, New York, 1960.

Sperelakis, N., Rubio, R. and Redick, J.: Sharp discontinuity in sarcomere lengths across intercalated disk of fibrillating cat hearts. *J. Ultrastruct. Res.* 30:503, 1970.

Wilcken, D. E. L., Brender, D., Shorey, C. D. and MacDonald, G. J.: Reserpine: Effect on structure of heart muscle. *Science* 157:1332, 1967.

Smooth Muscle

Caesar, R., Edwards, G. A. and Ruska, H.: Architecture and nerve supply of mammalian smooth muscle tissue. *J. Biophys. Biochem. Cytol.* 3:867, 1957.

Dewey, M. M. and Barr, L.: Intercellular connection between smooth muscle cells. The nexus. *Science* 137:670, 1962.

Garamvölgyi, N., Vizi, E. S. and Knoll, J.: The regular occurrence of thick filaments in stretched mammalian smooth muscle. *J. Ultrastruct. Res.* 34:135, 1971.

Lane, B. P.: Alterations in the cytologic detail of intestinal smooth muscle cells in various stages of contraction. *J. Cell Biol.* 27:199, 1965.

Osvaldo-Decima, L.: Smooth muscle in the ovary of the rat and monkey. *J. Ultrastruct. Res.* 29:218, 1970.

Panner, B. J. and Honig, C. R.: Filament ultrastructure and organization in vertebrate smooth muscle. Contraction hypothesis passed on localization of actin and myosin. *J. Cell Biol.* 35:303, 1967.

Ross, R. and Klebanoff, S. J.: Fine structural changes in uterine smooth muscle and fibroblasts in response to estrogen. *J. Cell Biol.* 32:155, 1967.

Yamauchi, H. and Burnstock, G.: Post-natal development of smooth muscle cells of the mouse vas deferens. A fine structural study. *J. Anat.* 104:1, 1969.

Myoneural Junction

Barrnett, R. J.: The fine structural localization of acetylcholinesterase at the myoneural junction. *J. Cell Biol.* 12:247, 1962.

Couteaux, R.: Motor end-plate structure. In *The Structure and Function of Muscle* (Bourne, G., ed.). Academic Press, New York, 1960.

Lentz, T. L.: Development of the neuromuscular junction. *J. Cell Biol.* 47:423, 1970.

Padykula, H. A. and Gauthier, G. F.: The ultrastructure of the neuromuscular junctions of mammalian red, white, and intermediate skeletal muscle fibers. *J. Cell Biol.* 46:27, 1970.

Salpeter, M. M.: Electron microscope radioautography as a quantitative tool in enzyme cytochemistry. The distribution of acetylcholinesterase at motor end plates of a vertebrate twitch muscle. *J. Cell Biol.* 32:379, 1967.

Nerve

Neuron

Babel, J.: *Ultrastructure of the Peripheral Nervous System.* C. V. Mosby Company, St. Louis, 1970.

Bodian, D.: The generalized vertebrate neuron. *Science 137:*323, 1962.

Duffy, P. E. and Tennyson, V. M.: Phase and electron microscopic observations of Lewy bodies and melanin granules in substantia nigra and locus caeruleus in Parkinson's disease. *J. Neuropath. Exp. Neurol. 24:*398, 1965.

Gonatas, N. K. and Goldensohn, E. S.: Unusual neocortical presynaptic terminals in a patient with convulsions, mental retardation and cortical blindness: An electron microscopic study. *J. Neuropath. Exp. Neurol. 24:*539, 1965.

Hamberger, A., Hansson, H. and Sjostrand, J.: Surface structure of isolated neurons. *J. Cell Biol. 47:*319, 1970.

Lojek, J. S. and Orlob, G. B.: Synaptic vesicles in electron micrographs of freeze-etched nerve terminals. *Science 164:*1405, 1969.

Moses, H. L., Beaver, D. L. and Ganote, C. E.: Electron microscopy of the trigeminal ganglion. 1. Comparative ultrastructure. *Arch. Path. 79:*541, 1965.

Samorajski, T., Ordy, J. M. and Keefe, J. R.: The fine structure of lipofuscin age pigment in the nervous system of aged mice. *J. Cell Biol. 26:*779, 1965.

Neuroglia

Duffell, D., Farber, L., Chou, S., Hartmann, J. F. and Nelson, E.: Electron microscopic observations on astrocytomas. *Amer. J. Path. 43:*539, 1963.

Fogelson, M. H., Gonatas, N. K., Rorke, L. B. and Spiro, A.: Oligodendroglial lamellar inclusions. *Arch. Neurol. 19:*150, 1968.

Luse, S. A.: Ultrastructure of reactive and neoplastic astrocytes. *Lab. Invest. 7:*401, 1958.

Lynn, J. A., Panopia, I. T., Martin, J. H., Shaw, M. L. and Race, G. J.: Ultrastructural evidence for astroglial histogenesis of the monstrocellular astrocytoma (so-called monstrocellular sarcoma of brain). *Cancer 22:*356, 1968.

Maxwell, D. S. and Kruger, L.: The fine structure of astrocytes in the cerebral cortex and their response to focal injury produced by heavy ionizing particles. *J. Cell Biol. 25*(Suppl.):141, 1965.

Peripheral Nerves

Bischoff, A. and Moor, H.: Ultrastructural differences between the myelin sheaths of peripheral nerve fibers and CNS white matter. *Z. Zellforsch. 81:*303, 1967.

Brannon, W., McCormick, W. and Lampert, P.: Axonal dystrophy in the gracile nucleus of man. *Acta Neuropath. 9:*1, 1967.

Cravioto, H.: The role of Schwann cells in the development of human peripheral nerves. *J. Ultrastruct. Res. 12:*634, 1965.

Gamble, H. J. and Eames, R. A.: An electron microscopic study of the connective tissue of the human peripheral nerve. *J. Anat. 98:*655, 1964.

Gamble, H. J.: Comparative electron-microscopic observations on the connective tissues of a peripheral nerve and a spinal nerve root in the rat. *J. Anat. 98:*17, 1964.

Gamble, H. J. and Breathnach, A. S.: An electron-microscopic study of human foetal peripheral nerves. *J. Anat. 99:*573, 1965.

Haftek, J. and Thomas, P. K.: Electron-microscope observations on the effects of localized crush injuries on the connective tissues of peripheral nerve. *J. Anat. 103:*233, 1968.

Lampert, P. W.: A comparative electron microscopic study of reactive, degenerating, regenerating, and dystrophic axons. *J. Neuropath. Exp. Neurol. 26:*345, 1967.

Rawlins, F. A. and Uzman, B. G.: Retardation of peripheral nerve myelination in mice treated with inhibitors of cholesterol biosynthesis. *J. Cell Biol. 46:*505, 1970.

Uga, S. and Ikui, H.: Membrane modification occurring between neurons and Schwann cells. *J. Electron Micr. 17:*155, 1968.

Webster, H.: The geometry of peripheral myelin sheaths during their formation and growth in rat sciatic nerves. *J. Cell Biol. 48:*348, 1971.

Cerebrum—Brain Stem

Adachi, M., Wallace, B. J., Schneck, L. and Volk, B. W.: Fine structure of spongy degeneration of the central nervous system (van Bogaert and Bertrand type). *J. Neuropath. Exp. Neurol. 25:*598, 1966.

Bodian, D.: An electron microscopic characterization of classes of synaptic vesicles by means of controlled aldehyde fixation. *J. Cell Biol. 44:*115, 1970.

Descarries, L. and Droz, B.: Intraneural distribution of exogenous norepinephrine in the central nervous system of the rat. *J. Cell Biol. 44:*385, 1970.

Gonatas, N. K.: Subacute sclerosing leucoencephalitis. Electron microscopic and cytochemical observations on a cerebral biopsy. *J. Neuropath. Exp. Neurol. 25:*177, 1966.

Gonatas, N. K., Baird, H. W. and Evangelista, I.: The fine structure of neocortical synapses in infantile amaurotic idiocy. *J. Neuropath. Exp. Neurol. 27:*39, 1968.

Misugi, K., Less, L. and Bradel, E. J.: Electron microscopic study of an ectopic pinealoma. *Acta Neuropath. 9:*346, 1967.

Waggener, J. D. and Beggs, J.: The membranous coverings of neural tissues: An electron microscopy study. *J. Neuropath. Exp. Neurol. 26:*412, 1967.

Wartenberg, H.: The mammalian pineal organ: Electron microscopic studies on the fine structure of pinealocytes, glial cells and on the perivascular compartment. *Z. Zellforsch. 86:*74, 1968.

Zu Rhein, G. M. and Chou, S. M.: Subacute sclerosing panencephalitis. Ultrastructural study of a brain biopsy. *Neurology 18:*146, 1968.

Cerebellum

Herndon, R. M.: The fine structure of the rat cerebellum. II. The stellate neurons, granular cells and glia. *J. Cell Biol. 23:*277, 1964.

Wallace, B. J., Schneck, L., Kaplan, J. and Volk, B. W.: Fine structure of the cerebellum of children with lipidoses. *Arch. Path. 80:*466, 1965.

Ganglion

Adachi, M., Volk, B. W., Schneck, L. and Torii, J.: Fine structure of the myenteric plexus in various lipidoses. *Arch. Path. 87:*228, 1969.

Dixon, J. S.: The fine structure of parasympathetic nerve cells in the otic ganglia of the rabbit. *Anat. Rec. 156:*239, 1966.

Gunn, M.: Histological and histochemical observations on the myenteric and submucous plexuses of mammals. *J. Anat. 102:*223, 1968.

Pick, J.: Fine structure of nerve terminals in the human gut. *Anat. Rec. 159:*131, 1967.

Tennyson, V. M. and Brzin, M.: The appearance of acetylcholinesterase in the dorsal root neuroblast of the rabbit embryo. *J. Cell Biol. 46:*64, 1970.

Watari, N.: Fine structure of nervous elements in the pancreas of some vertebrates. *Z. Zellforsch. 85:*291, 1968.

Yates, R. D., Chen, I. and Duncan, D.: Effects of sinus nerve stimulation on carotid body glomus cells. *J. Cell Biol.* 46:544, 1970.

Nerve Endings

Cauna, N.: Structure of digital touch receptors. *Acta Anat.* 32:1, 1958.

Cauna, N. and Ross, L. L.: The fine structure of Meissner's touch corpuscles of human fingers. *J. Biophys. Biochem. Cytol.* 8:467, 1960.

Henry Ford Hospital: *Pain.* Little Brown and Company, Boston, 1966.

Patrizi, G. and Munger, B. L.: The cytology of encapsulated nerve endings in the rat penis. *J. Ultrastruct. Res.* 13:500, 1965.

Pease, D. C. and Pallie, W.: Electron microscopy of digital tactile corpuscles and small cutaneous nerves. *J. Ultrastruct. Res.* 2:352, 1959.

Circulatory System

Arteries

Ahmed, M. M.: The fine structure of endothelium in coronary arterioles. *Acta Anat.* 69:327, 1968.

Berman, H. J. and Siggens, G. R.: Neurogenic factors in the microvascular system. *Fed. Proc.* 27:1384, 1968.

Daoud, A. S., Jones, R. and Scott, R. F.: Dietary-induced atherosclerosis in miniature swine. 2. Electron microscopy observations: Characteristics of endothelial and smooth muscle cells in the proliferative lesions and elsewhere in the aorta. *Exp. Molec. Path.* 8:263, 1968.

French, J. E., Jennings, M. A. and Florey, H. W.: Morphological studies on atherosclerosis in swine. *Ann. N. Y. Acad. Sci.* 127:780, 1965.

Fyfe, F. W., Gillman, T. and Onesin, I. B.: A combined quantitative chemical, light, and electron microscope study of aortic development in normal and nitrite-treated mice. *Ann. N. Y. Acad. Sci.* 149:607, 1968.

Haust, M. D., More, R. H., Bencosme, S. A. and Balis, J. U.: Elastogenesis in human aorta: An electron microscopic study. *Exp. Molec. Path.* 4:508, 1965.

Hayes, J. R.: Histological changes in constricted arteries and arterioles. *J. Anat.* 101:343, 1967.

Hoff, H. F. and Gottlob, R.: A fine structure study of injury to the endothelial cells of the rabbit abdominal aorta by various stimuli. *Angiology* 18:440, 1967.

Jaffé, D., Manning, M. and Hartroft, W. S.: Coronary arteries in the earlier decades of man. *Fed. Proc.* 27:575, 1968.

Lang, E. R. and Kidd, M.: Electron microscopy of human cerebral aneurysms. *J. Neurosurg.* 22:554, 1965.

Lever, J. D., Ahmed, M. and Irvine, G.: Neuromuscular and intercellular relationship in the coronary arterioles. A morphological and quantitative study by light and electron microscopy. *J. Anat.* 99:829, 1965.

Pease, D. C. and Molinari, S.: Electron microscopy of muscular arteries: Pial vessels of the cat and monkey. *J. Ultrastruct. Res.* 3:447, 1960.

Rees, P. M.: Electron microscopical observations on the architecture of the carotid arterial walls, with special reference to the sinus portion. *J. Anat.* 103:35, 1968.

Rhodin, J. A. G.: Fine structure of vascular walls in mammals with special reference to smooth muscle component. *Physiol. Rev.* 42:447, 1962.

Verity, M. A. and Bevan, J. A.: Fine structural study of the terminal effector plexus, neuromuscular and intermuscular relationships in the pulmonary artery. *J. Anat.* *103*:49, 1968.

Veins
Wood, J. E.: *The Veins: Normal and Abnormal Function.* Little, Brown and Company, Boston, 1965.

Capillaries
Abramson, D. I. (ed.): *Blood Vessels and Lymphatics.* Academic Press, New York, 1962.

Barer, R.: The ultrastructure of small blood vessels of the posterior pituitary gland in relation to neurosecretion. *Bibl. Anat.* *7*:304, 1965.

Bennett, H. S., Luft, J. H. and Hampton, J. C.: Morphological classifications of vertebrate blood capillaries. *Amer. J. Physiol.* *196*:381, 1959.

Bruns, R. R. and Palade, G. E.: Studies on blood capillaries. I. General organization of blood capillaries in muscle. *J. Cell Biol.* *37*:244, 1968.

Cohen, A. S.: Amyloidosis. *New Eng. J. Med.* *277*:522, 1967.

Cotran, R. S., La Gattuta, M. and Majno, G.: Studies on inflammation fate of intramural vascular deposits induced by histamine. *Amer. J. Path.* *47*:1045, 1965.

Karnovsky, M. J. and Cotran, R. S.: The intercellular passage of exogenous peroxidase across endothelium and mesothelium. *Anat. Rec.* *154*:365, 1966.

Larsson, O.: Studies of small vessels in patients with diabetes. *Acta Med. Scand. Suppl.* *480*:5, 1967.

Majno, G. and Palade, G. E.: Studies on inflammation. 1. The effect of histamine and serotonin on vascular permeability: An electron microscopic study. *J. Biophys. Biochem. Cytol.* *11*:571, 1961.

Majno, G., Shea, S. M. and Leventhal, M.: Endothelial contraction induced by histamine-type mediators. *J. Cell Biol.* *42*:647, 1969.

Uracko, R. and Benditt, E. P.: Capillary basal lamina thickening. *J. Cell Biol.* *47*:281, 1970.

Lymphoid System

Lymphoid Cells
Epstein, M. A. and Achong, B. G.: Fine structural organization of human lymphoblasts of a tissue culture strain (EBI) from Burkit's lymphoma. *J. Nat. Cancer Inst.* *34*:241, 1965.

Heiniger, H. J., Riedwyl, H., Giger, H., Sordat, B. and Cottier, H.: Ultrastructural differences between thymic and lymph node small lymphocytes of mice: Nucleolar size and cytoplasmic volume. *Blood* *30*:288, 1967.

Johnson, F. R. and Roberts, K. B.: The growth and division of human small lymphocytes in tissue culture: An electron microscopic study. *J. Anat.* *98*:303, 1964.

Storb, U., Chambers, V., Storb, R. and Weiser, R. S.: Antibody-carrying cells in the immune response. 2. Ultrastructure of "rosette"-forming cells. *J. Reticuloendothel. Soc.* *4*:69, 1967.

Tokuyasu, K., Madden, S. C. and Zeldis, L. J.: Fine structural alterations of interphase nuclei of lymphocytes stimulated to growth activity in vitro. *J. Cell Biol.* *39*:630, 1968.

Uzman, B. G., Foley, G. E., Farber, S., and Lazarus, H.: Morphologic variations in human leukemic lymphoblasts (CCRF-CEM cells) after long-term culture and exposure to chemotherapeutic agents. A study with the electron microscope. *Cancer 19*:1725, 1966.

Lymph Nodes

Djaldetti, M., Sandbank, U. and Danon, D.: Effect of Echis colorata envenomation on circulating lymphocytes and lymph nodes of the guinea pig. An electron microscopic study. *Rev. Franc. Etud. Clin. Biol. 12*:55, 1967.

Dobbins, W. O. and Rollins, E. L.: Intestinal mucosal lymphatic permeability: An electron microscopic study of endothelial vesicles and cell junctions. *J. Ultrastruct. Res. 33*:29, 1970.

Moe, R. E.: Electron microscopic appearance of the parenchyma of lymph nodes. *Amer. J. Anat. 114*:341, 1964.

Smith, E. B., White, D. C., Hartsock, R. J., and Dixon, A. C.: Acute ultrastructural effects of 500 roentgens on the lymph node of the mouse. *Amer. J. Path. 50*:159, 1967.

Wyllie, J. C.: Electron microscopy of cellular changes observed in lymph nodes of the guinea pig during the development of contact sensitivity. *Rev. Canad. Biol. 25*:195, 1966.

Yamori, T. and Mori, Y.: Electron microscopic observation of reticuloendothelial system. *Tohoku J. Exp. Med. 81*:330, 1964.

Spleen

Berendsen, P. B. and Telford, I. R.: A light and electron microscopic study of Kurloff bodies in the blood and spleen of the guinea pig. *Anat. Rec. 156*:107, 1966.

Edwards, V. D. and Simon, G. T.: Ultrastructural aspects of red cell destruction in the normal rat spleen. *J. Ultrastruct. Res. 33*:187, 1970.

Lennert, K. and Harms, D.: *The Spleen.* Springer-Verlag, Berlin, 1970.

Seki, M., Sekiyama, S. and Yoneyama, T.: Electron microscopic studies on the spleen of normal mouse and its morphological changes after total body irradiation. *J. Radiat. Res. 5*:183, 1964.

Simic, M. M.: Morphologic variations in the locally irradiated spleen related to the immune response. *J. Cell Physiol. 67*(Suppl.):129, 1966.

Swartzendruber, D. C. and Hanna, M. G.: Electron microscopic autoradiography of germinal center cells in mouse spleen. *J. Cell Biol. 25*:109, 1965.

Szakal, A. K. and Hanna, M. G.: The ultrastructure of antigen localization and virus-like particles in mouse spleen germinal centers. *Exp. Molec. Path. 8*:75, 1968.

Thymus

Blackburn, W. R. and Gordon, D. S.: The thymic remnant in thymic alymphoplasia. Light and electron microscopic studies. *Arch. Path. 84*:363, 1967.

Ghossein, N. A., Azar, H. A. and Williams, J.: Local irradiation of the thymus. Histological changes with observations on circulating lymphocytes and serum protein fractions in adult mice. *Amer. J. Path. 43*:369, 1963.

Kameya, T. and Watanabe, Y.: Electron microscopic observations on human thymus and thymoma. *Acta Path. Jap. 15*:223, 1965.

Kohnen, P. and Weiss, L.: An electron microscopic study of thymic corpuscles in the guinea pig and the mouse. *Anat. Rec. 148*:29, 1964.

Murray, R. G., Murray, A. and Pizzo, A.: The fine structure of the thymocytes of young rats. *Anat. Rec. 151*:17, 1965.

Pinkel, D.: Ultrastructure of human fetal thymus. *Amer. J. Dis. Child. 115:222,* 1968.

Sebuwufu, P. H.: Ultrastructure of human fetal thymic cilia. *J. Ultrastruct. Res. 24:171,* 1968.

Sebuwufu, P. H.: Crystalline inclusions in normal primate thymoblasts. *Nature 218:980,* 1968.

Vethamany, V. G. and Engelbert, V. E.: An electron microscopic study of eosinophil formation in the rabbit thymus. *Haemat. Lat. 11:93,* 1968.

Endocrine Glands

Pituitary

Conklin, J. L.: The identification of acidophilic cells in the human pars distalis. *Anat. Rec. 156:347,* 1966.

Dekler, A.: Pituitary basophils of the Syrian hamster: An electron microscope investigation. *Anat. Rec. 158:351,* 1967.

Foncin, J. F. and Le Beau, J.: Cellules de castration et cellules FSH dans l'hypophyse humaine vues au microscope electronique. *J. Microscopie 5:523,* 1966.

Green, J. D.: Electron microscopy of the anterior pituitary. In *The Pituitary Gland* (Harris, G. W. and Donovan, B. T., eds.). Butterworth, London and Washington, 1966.

Herlant, M.: The cells of the adenohypophysis and their functional significance. *Int. Rev. Cytol. 17:299,* 1964.

Kobayashi, Y.: Functional morphology of the pars intermedia of the rat hypophysis as revealed with the electron microscope. 2. Correlation of the pars intermedia with the hypophyseo-adrenal axis. *Z. Zellforsch. 68:11,* 1965.

Kurosumi, K.: Functional classification of cell types of the anterior pituitary gland accomplished by electron microscopy. *Arch. Histol. Jap. 29:329,* 1968.

Lederis, K.: Electron microscopy of the human anterior pituitary. *Acta Endocr. 100(Suppl.):159,* 1965.

Lederis, K.: An electron microscopical study of the human neurohypophysis. *Z. Zellforsch. 65:847,* 1965.

Monroe, B. G.: A comparative study of the ultrastructure of the median eminence, infundibular stem and neural lobe of the hypophysis of the rat. *Z. Zellforsch. 76:405,* 1967.

Potvliege, P. R.: Effects of estrogen on pituitary morphology in estrogen-treated rats. An electron microscopic study. *Anat. Rec. 160:595,* 1968.

Schelin, U.: Chromophobe and acidophil adenomas of the human pituitary gland. A light and electron microscopic study. *Acta Microbiol. Scand. 158(Suppl.):1,* 1962.

van Oordt, P.: Nomenclature of the hormone-producing cells in the adenohypophysis. A report of the international committee for nomenclature of the adenohypophysis. *Gen. Comp. Endocr. 5:131,* 1965.

Voitkevich, A. A.: Differentiation of basophil and oxyphil cells in the pituitary. *Arkh. Anat. 49(9):3,* 1965.

Yoshimura, F. and Harumiya, K.: Electron microscopy of the anterior lobe of pituitary in normal and castrated rats. *Endocr. Jap. 12:119,* 1965.

Zambrano, D.: Ultrastructural changes of the neurohypophysis of the rat after castration. *Z. Zellforsch. 86:14,* 1968.

Suprarenal

Brenner, R. M.: Fine structure of adrenocortical cells in adult male rhesus monkeys. *Amer. J. Anat. 119*:429, 1966.

Dietert, S. E.: An ultrastructural and biochemical study of the effects of three inhibitors of cholesterol biosynthesis upon murine adrenal gland and testis. Histochemical evidence for a lysosome response. *J. Cell Biol. 40*:44, 1969.

Elfvin, L. G.: The development of the secretory granules in the rat adrenal medulla. *J. Ultrastruct. Res. 17*:45, 1967.

Elfvin, L. G., Appelgren, L. E. and Ullberg, S.: High-resolution autoradiography of the adrenal medulla after injection of tritiated dihydroxyphenylalanine (Dopa). *J. Ultrastruct. Res. 14*:277, 1966.

Friend, D. S. and Bassil, G. E.: Osmium staining of endoplasmic reticulum and mitochondria in the rat adrenal cortex. *J. Cell Biol. 46*:252, 1970.

Hoshino, M.: "Polysome lamellae complex" in the adenoma cells of the human adrenal cortex. *J. Ultrastruct. Res. 27*:205, 1969.

Kahri, A. I.: Effects of actinomycin D and puromycin on the ACTH-induced ultrastructural transformation of mitochondria of cortical cells of rat adrenals in tissue culture. *J. Cell Biol. 36*:181, 1968.

Mori, M. and Onoe, T.: Electron microscopic study on capillary endothelial cells of the adrenal cortex. *Tohoku J. Exp. Med. 93*:301, 1967.

Moses, H. L., Davis, W. W., Rosenthal, A. S. and Garren, L. D.: Adrenal cholesterol: Localization by electron-microscope autoradiography. *Science 163*:1203, 1969.

Nickerson, P. A., Skelton, F. R., and Molteni, A.: Observation of filaments in the adrenal of androgen-treated rats. *J. Cell Biol. 47*:277, 1970.

Rhodin, J. A. G.: The ultrastructure of the adrenal cortex of the rat under normal and experimental conditions. *J. Ultrastruct. Res. 34*:23, 1971.

Schardein, J. L., Patton, G. R. and Lucas, J. A.: The microscopy of "brown degeneration" in the adrenal gland of the mouse. *Anat. Rec. 159*:291, 1967.

Sheridan, M. N. and Belt, W. D.: Fine structure of the guinea pig adrenal cortex. *Anat. Rec. 149*:73, 1964.

Williams, V. and Morriss, F.: Formaldehyde-induced fluorescences as a means for differentiating epinephrine cells from norepinephrine cells in adrenal medulla. *Stain Techn. 45*:205, 1970.

Wood, J. G.: Identification of and observations on epinephrine and norepinephrine containing cells in the adrenal medulla. *Amer. J. Anat. 112*:285, 1963.

Yates, R. D., Wood, J. G. and Dungan, D.: Phase and electron microscopic observations on two cell types in the adrenal medulla of the Syrian hamster. *Texas Rep. Biol. Med. 20*:494, 1962.

Zelander, T.: Endocrine organs: The adrenal gland. In *Electron Microscopic Anatomy* (Kurtz, S. M., ed.). Academic Press, New York, 1964.

Pancreas

Bencosme, S. A., Allen, R. A. and Latta, H.: Functioning pancreatic islet cell tumors studied electron microscopically. *Amer. J. Path. 42*:1, 1963.

Boquist, L.: Alloxan administration in the Chinese hamster. 2. Ultrastructural study of degeneration and subsequent regeneration of the pancreatic islet tissue. *Virchow Arch. Abt. B. Zellpathol. 1*:169, 1968.

Björkman, N., Hellerström, C., Hellman, B. and Petersson, B.: The cell types in the endocrine pancreas of the human fetus. *Z. Zellforsch. 72:425, 1966.*

Caramia, F., Munger, B. L. and Lacy, P. E.: The ultrastructural basis for the identification of cell types in the pancreatic islets. 1. Guinea pig. *Z. Zellforsch. 67:533, 1965.*

Findlay, J. A., Gill, J. R., Irvine, E., Lever, J. D. and Randle, P. J.: Cytology of B-cells in rabbit pancreas pieces incubated in vitro: Effects of glucose and tolbutamide. *Diabetologia 4:150, 1968.*

Gomez-Acebo, J.: Fine structure of the A and D cells of the rabbit endocrine pancreas in vivo and incubated in vitro. I. Mechanism of secretion of the A cells. *J. Cell Biol. 36:33, 1968.*

Lacy, P. E.: Electron microscopy of the beta cell of the pancreas. *Amer. J. Med. 31:851, 1961.*

Lehy, T. and Zeitoun, X.: Influence of fixatives on the metachromatic reaction to toluidine blue at pH 5; A_1 and A_2 cells of human endocrine pancreas. *Stain Techn. 45:63, 1970.*

Like, A. A.: The ultrastructure of the islets of Langerhans in man. *Lab. Invest. 16:937, 1967.*

Logothetopoulos, J., Davidson, J. K., Haist, R. E. and Best, C. H.: Degranulation of beta cells and loss of pancreatic insulin after infusions of insulin antibody or glucose. *Diabetes 14:493, 1965.*

Machino, M.: On the substructures of secretory granules of the chick beta islet cell. *J. Ultrastruct. Res. 31:199, 1970.*

Munger, B. L., Caramia, F. and Lacy, P. E.: The ultrastructural basis for the identification of cell types in the pancreatic islets. 2. Rabbit, dog and opossum. *Z. Zellforsch. 67:776, 1965.*

Spooner, B. S., Walther, B. T. and Rutter, W. J.: The development of the dorsal and ventral mammalian pancreas in vivo and vitro. *J. Cell Biol. 47:235, 1970.*

Wellmann, K. F., Brancato, P., Lazarus, S. S. and Volk, B. W.: Rabbit beta cell ultrastructure and insulin radio-immunoassay in experimental subdiabetes. *Arch. Path. 84:251, 1967.*

Thyroid

Braunstein, H., Stephens, C. L. and Givson, R. L.: Secretory granules in medullary carcinoma of the thyroid. *Arch. Path. 85:306, 1968.*

Ekholm, R.: Thyroglobulin biosynthesis in the rat thyroid. *J. Ultrastruct. Res. 20:103, 1967.*

Ekholm, R. and Ericson, L. E.: The ultrastructure of the parafollicular cells of the thyroid gland in the rat. *J. Ultrastruct. Res. 23:378, 1968.*

Ericson, L. E.: Subcellular localization of 5-hydroxytryptamine in the para follicular cells of the mouse thyroid gland. An autoradiographic study. *J. Ultrastruct. Res. 31:162, 1970.*

Lupulescu, A. and Petrovici, A.: *Ultrastructure of the Thyroid Gland.* M. D. Anderson Tumor Institute, Houston, 1968.

Pantić, V., Pavlović-Hournac, M. and Rappaport, L.: Relation entre l'ultrastructure des cultures et des greffes de glandes thyroides de rats et leur pouvoir de synthèse de la thyroglobuline. *J. Ultrastruct. Res. 31:37, 1970.*

Matsuzawa, T. and Kurosumi, K.: Morphological changes in the parafollicular cells of the rat thyroid glands after administration of calcium shown by electron microscopy. *Nature 213:926, 1967.*

Neve, P.: Ultrastructure des cellules folliculaires d'une thyroide humaine normale. *J. Microscopie.* 4:811, 1965.

Neve, P., Rodesch, F. R. and Dumont, J. E.: Electron microscopy of isolated sheep thyroid cells. *Exp. Cell Res.* 51:68, 1968.

Seljelid, R.: Endocytosis in thyroid follicle cells. I. Structure and significance of different types of single membrane-limited vacuoles and bodies. *J. Ultrastruct. Res.* 17:195, 1967.

Sobel, H. J.: Electron microscopy of I-irradiated thyroid. *Arch. Path.* 78:53, 1964.

Themann, H., Andrada, J. A., Rose, N. R., Andrada, E. C. and Witebsky, E.: Experimental thyroiditis in the rhesus monkey. 5. Electron microscopic investigations. *Clin. Exp. Immun.* 3:491, 1968.

Wetzel, B. K., Spicer, S. S. and Wollman, S. H.: Changes in fine structure and acid phosphatase localization in rat thyroid cells following thyrotropin administration. *J. Cell Biol.* 25:593, 1965.

Young, B. A.: Cell types in the mammalian thyroid gland. *Int. Rev. Gen. Exp. Zool.* 3:396, 1968.

Parathyroid

Capen, C. C. and Rowland, G. N.: The ultrastructure of the parathyroid glands of young cats. *Anat. Rec.* 162:327, 1968.

Gaillard, P. J., Talmage, R. V. and Budy, A. M. (eds.): *The Parathyroid Glands.* University of Chicago Press, Chicago, 1965.

Lever, J. D.: Fine structural organization of the human and rat parathyroid glands. In *The Parathyroid Glands* (Gaillard, P. J., Talmage, R. V. and Budy, A. M., eds.). University of Chicago Press, Chicago, 1965.

Mazzocchi, G., Meneghelli, V. and Frasson, F.: The human parathyroid glands: An optical and electron microscopic study. *Sperimentale* 117:383, 1967.

Nakagami, K., Yamazaki, Y. and Tsunoda, Y.: An electron microscopic study of the human fetal parathyroid gland. *Z. Zellforsch.* 85:89, 1968.

Roth, S. I., Au, W. Y., Kunin, A. S., Krane, S. M. and Raisz, L. G.: Effect of dietary deficiency in vitamin D, calcium, and phosphorus on the ultrastructure of the rat parathyroid gland. *Amer. J. Path.* 53:631, 1968.

Male Reproductive System

Testis—Interstitial

Christensen, A. K. and Fawcett, D. W.: The normal fine structure of opossum testicular interstitial cells. *J. Biophys. Biochem. Cytol.* 9:653, 1961.

Fawcett, D. W. and Burgos, M. H.: Observations on the cytomorphosis of the germinal and interstitial cells of the human testis. In *Ciba Foundation Colloquia on Aging.* J. & A. Churchill, London, 1956.

Fawcett, D. W. and Burgos, M. H.: Studies on the fine structure of the mammalian testis. II. The human interstitial tissue. *Amer. J. Anat.* 107:245, 1960.

Hatakeyama, S.: A study on the interstitial cells of the human testis, especially on their fine-structural pathology. *Acta Path. Jap.* 15:155, 1965.

Kretser, D. M. D.: The fine structure of the testicular interstitial cells in men of normal androgenic status. *Z. Zellforsch.* 80:594, 1967.

Schneider, N. P., Stephens, R. J. and Gardner, W. U.: Viral inclusions and other cytoplasmic components in a Leydig cell murine tumor: An electron microscopic study. *Int. J. Cancer* 3:155, 1968.

Testis

Clermont, Y.: The cycle of the seminiferous epithelium in man. *Amer. J. Anat. 112:35*, 1963.

Heller, C. G. and Clermont, Y.: Kinetics of the germinal epithelium in man. *Recent Progr. Hormone Res. 20:545*, 1964.

Matano, Y.: Ultrastructural study on human binucleate spermatids. *J. Ultrastruct. Res. 34:123*, 1971.

Ross, M. H. and Long, I. R.: Contractile cells in human seminiferous tubules. *Science 153:1271*, 1966.

Sohval, A. R., Suzuki, Y., Gabrilove, J. L. and Churg, J.: Ultrastructure of crystalloids in spermatogonia and Sertoli cells of normal human testis. *J. Ultrastruct. Res. 34:83*, 1971.

Spermatogenesis and Spermiogenesis

Bedford, J. M.: Observations on the fine structure of spermatozoa of the Bush baby (Galago senegalensis), the African green monkey (Cercopithecus aethiops) and man. *Amer. J. Anat. 121:443*, 1967.

Clermont, Y. and Leblond, C. P.: Spermiogenesis of man, monkey, ram and other mammals as shown by the "periodic acid-Schiff" technique. *Amer. J. Anat. 96:229*, 1955.

Fawcett, D. W.: The anatomy of the mammalian spermatozoan with particular references to the guinea pig. *Z. Zellforsch. 67:279*, 1965.

Pedersen, H.: Observations on the axial filament complex of the human spermatozoon. *J. Ultrastruct. Res. 33:451*, 1970.

Phillips, D. M.: Development of spermatozoa in the wooly opossum with special reference to the shaping of the sperm head. *J. Ultrastruct. Res. 33:369*, 1970.

Rattner, J. B. and Brinkley, B. R.: Ultrastructure of spermiogenesis. *J. Ultrastruct. Res. 32:316*, 1970.

Vitale-Calpe, R. and Burgos, M. H.: The mechanism of spermiation in the hamster. *J. Ultrastruct. Res. 31:381*, 1970.

Prostate

Fisher, E. R. and Jeffrey, W.: Ultrastructure of human normal and neoplastic prostate. *Amer. J. Clin. Path. 44:119*, 1965.

Györkey, F.: The appearance of acid phosphatase in human prostate gland. *Lab. Invest. 13:105*, 1964.

Härkönen, M., Niemi, M. and Söderholm, U.: Histochemistry of rat prostatic complex. *Lab. Invest. 13:45*, 1964.

Riva, A.: Ultrastruttura dell'epitelio delle vescichette seminali umane. *Arch. Ital. Anat. Embriol. 72(Suppl.):113*, 1967.

Female Reproductive System

Ovary

Baca, M. and Zamboni, L.: The fine structure of human follicular oocytes. *J. Ultrastruct. Res. 19:354*, 1967.

Baker, T. G. and Franchi, L. L.: The fine structure of oogonia and oocytes in human ovaries. *J. Cell Sci. 2:213*, 1967.

Espey, L. L.: Ultrastructure of the apex of the rabbit graafian follicle during the ovulatory process. *Endocrinology 81*:267, 1967.

Franceschini, M. P., Santoro, A. and Motta, P.: L'ultrastruttura delle cellule della granulosa nelle varie fasi di maturazione del follicolo ooforo (Richerche in Lepus cuniculus, Linn.). *Boll. Soc. Ital. Biol. Sper. 41*:1, 1965.

Green, J. A. and Maqueo, M.: Ultrastructure of the human ovary. 1. The luteal cell during the menstrual cycle. *J. Obstet. Gynec. 92*:946, 1965.

Hadek, R.: *Mammalian Fertilization: An Atlas of Ultrastructure.* Academic Press, New York and London, 1969.

Hertig, A. T. and Adams, E. C.: Studies on the human oocyte and its follicle. 1. Ultrastructural and histochemical observations on the primordial follicle stage. *J. Cell Biol. 34*:647, 1967.

Hertig, A. T.: The primary human oocyte: Some observations on the fine structure of Balbiani's vitelline body and the origin of the annulate lamellae. *Amer. J. Anat. 122*:107, 1968.

Hope, J.: The fine structure of the developing follicle of the Rhesus ovary. *J. Ultrastruct. Res. 12*:592, 1965.

Huebner, E. and Anderson, E.: The effects of vinblastine sulfate on the microtubular organization of the ovary of Rhodnius prolixus. *J. Cell Biol. 46*:191, 1970.

Kempson, R. L.: Ultrastructure of ovarian stromal cell tumors. Sertoli-Leydig cell tumor and lipid cell tumor. *Arch. Path. 86*:492, 1968.

Maruffo, C. A.: Zona pellucida of Rhesus monkey ovum after gonadotropin stimulation. *Science 157*:1313, 1967.

Solari, A. J. and Tres, L. L.: The ultrastructure of the human sex vesicle. *Chromosoma 22*:16, 1967.

Toker, C.: Ultrastructure of a granulosa cell tumor. *Amer. J. Obstet. Gynec. 100*:388, 1968.

Toker, C.: Theca cell tumor. *Amer. J. Obstet. Gynec. 100*:779, 1968.

Zamboni, L., Mishell, D. R., Bell, J. H. and Baca, M.: Fine structure of the human ovum in the pronuclear stage. *J. Cell Biol. 30*:579, 1966.

Zamboni, L. and Gondos, B.: Intercellular bridges and synchronization of germ cell differentiation during oogenesis in the rabbit. *J. Cell Biol. 36*:276, 1968.

Uterus—Cervix—Vagina

Ashworth, C. T., Stembridge, V. A. and Luibel, F. J.: A study of basement membranes of normal epithelium, carcinoma in situ and invasive carcinoma of uterine cervix utilizing electron microscopy and histochemical methods. *Acta Cytol. 5*:369, 1961.

Caudros, A. and Cooper, R. A.: Ultrastructure of spontaneous vaginal keratinization in hanging-drop organ culture (Balb/cCrgl mice). *Z. Zellforsch. 84*:429, 1968.

Dessouky, D. A.: Electron microscopic studies of the myometrium of the guinea pig. *Amer. J. Obstet. Gynec. 100*:30, 1968.

Hando, T., Okada, D. M. and Zamboni, L.: Atypical cilia in human endometrium. *J. Cell Biol. 39*:475, 1968.

Laguens, R. P., Lagrutta, J., Koch, O. R. and Quijano, F.: Fine structure of human endocervical epithelium. *Amer. J. Obstet. Gynec. 98*:773, 1967.

Shingleton, H. M., Richart, R. M., Wiener, J. and Spiro, D.: Human cervical intraepithelial neoplasia. Fine structure of dysplasia and carcinoma in situ. *Cancer Res. 28*:695, 1968.

Wynn, R. M.: Intrauterine devices: Effects on ultrastructure of human endometrium. *Science 156:*1508, 1967.

Wynn, R. M. and Harris, J. A.: Ultrastructure of trophoblast and endometrium in invasive hydatidiform mole (chorioadenoma destruens). *Amer. J. Obstet. Gynec. 99:*1125, 1967.

Placenta
Ashley, C. A.: Study of the human placenta with the electron microscope. *Arch. Path. 80:*377, 1965.

Baranova, E. I.: Cytochemical investigation of decidual cells of human placenta. *Arkh. Anat. 69*(11):35, 1965.

Boyd, J. D., Hamilton, W. J. and Boyd, C. A. R.: The surface of the syncytium of the human chorionic villus. *J. Anat. 102:*553, 1968.

Davies, J. and Glasser, S. R.: Light and electron microscopic observations on a human placenta 2 weeks after fetal death. *Amer. J. Obstet. Gynec. 98:*1111, 1967.

Hertig, A. T.: Human trophoblast: Normal and abnormal. *Amer. J. Clin. Path. 47*(3):249, 1967.

Knoth, M.: Ultrastructure of chorionic villi from a four-somite human embryo. *J. Ultrastruct. Res. 25:*423, 1968.

Ruffolo, R., Benirschke, K., Covington, H. I. and Munro, A. B.: Electron microscopic study of the "X-cells" in septal cysts of the human placenta. *Amer. J. Obstet. Gynec. 99:*1147, 1967.

Thomas, C. E.: The ultrastructure of human amnion epithelium. *J. Ultrastruct. Res. 13:*65, 1965.

Wynn, R. M. and French, G. L.: Comparative ultrastructure of the mammalian amnion. *Amer. J. Obstet. Gynec. 31:*759, 1968.

Mammary Gland
Mills, E. S. and Topper, Y. J.: Mammary alveolar epithelial cells: Effect of hydrocortisone on ultrastructure. *Science 165:*1127, 1969.

Mills, E. S. and Topper, Y. J.: Some ultrastructural effects of insulin, hydrocortisone, and prolactin on mammary gland explants. *J. Cell Biol. 44:*310, 1970.

Nemanic, M. K. and Pitelka, D. R.: A scanning electron microscope study of the lactating mammary gland. *J. Cell Biol. 48:*410, 1971.

Oral Glands

Doyle, L. E., Lynn, J. A., Panopio, I. T. and Crass, G.: Ultrastructure of the chondroid regions of benign mixed tumor of salivary gland. *Cancer 22:*225, 1968.

Fukushima, M.: An electron microscopic study of human salivary gland tumors—pleomorphic adenoma and adenoid cystic carcinoma. *Bull. Tokyo Med. Dent. Univ. 15:*387, 1968.

Hand, A. R.: Nerve-acinar cell relationships in the rat parotid gland. *J. Cell Biol. 47:*540, 1970.

Hand, A. R.: The fine structure of Von Ebner's gland of the rat. *J. Cell Biol. 44:*340, 1970.

Redman, R. S. and Sreebny, L. M.: Proliferative behavior of differentiating cells in the developing rat parotid gland. *J. Cell Biol. 46:*81, 1970.

Strum, J. M. and Karnovsky, M. J.: Ultrastructural localization of peroxidase in sub-maxillary acinar cells. *J. Ultrastruct. Res. 31:323, 1970.*

Tandler, B. and Shipkey, F. H.: Ultrastructure of Warthin's tumor. 1. Mitochondria. *J. Ultrastruct. Res. 11:292, 1964.*

Tandler, B.: Ultrastructure of the human submaxillary gland. 3. Myoepithelium. *Z. Zellforsch. 68:852, 1965.*

Tandler, B. and Ross, L. L.: Observations of nerve terminals in human labial salivary glands. *J. Cell Biol. 42:339, 1969.*

Tapp, R. L.: The ultrastructure of watery vacuoles in the submandibular gland of the rat. *J. Roy. Micr. Soc. 88:1, 1967.*

Welsh, R. A. and Meyer, A. T.: Mixed tumors of human salivary gland. Histogenesis. *Arch. Path. 85:433, 1968.*

Digestive System

Stomach

Adkins, R. B., Ende, N. and Gobbel, W. G.: A correlation of parietal cell activity with ultrastructural alterations. *Surgery 62:1059, 1967.*

Elliott, R. L. and Guillen, R.: Gastric biopsies. An ultrastructural study with special reference to pernicious anemia. *Arch. Path. 77:258, 1964.*

Helander, H. F.: Early effect of x-irradiation on the ultrastructure of gastric fundus glands. *Radiat. Res. 26:244, 1965.*

Johnson, F. R. and Young, B. A.: Undifferentiated cells in gastric mucosa. *J. Anat. 101:617, 1967.*

Pfeiffer, C. J.: Surface topology of the stomach in man and the laboratory ferret. *J. Ultrastruct. Res. 33:252, 1970.*

Rosa, F.: Ultrastructure of the fundic region of the human stomach in the resting state. *Acta Cient. Venez. 16:58, 1965.*

Rubin, W.: Enzyme cytochemistry of gastric parietal cells at a fine structure level. *J. Cell Biol. 42:332, 1969.*

Solcia, E., Vassallo, G. and Sampietro, R.: Endocrine cells in the antro-pyloric mucosa of the stomach. *Z. Zellforsch. 81:474, 1967.*

Small Intestine

Behnke, O. and Moe, H.: An electron microscopic study of mature and differentiating Paneth cells in the rats, especially of their endoplasmic reticulum and lysosomes. *J. Cell Biol. 22:633, 1964.*

Bennet, G. and Leblond, C. P.: Formation of cell coat material for the whole surface of columnar cells in the rat small intestine, as visualized by radioautography with L-fucose-[3]H. *J. Cell Biol. 46:409, 1970.*

Brunser, O. and Luft, J. H.: Fine structure of the apex of absorptive cells from rat small intestine. *J. Ultrastruct. Res. 31:291, 1970.*

Cardell, R. R., Badenhausen, S. and Porter, K. R.: Intestinal triglyceride absorption in the rat. An electron microscopical study. *J. Cell Biol. 34:123, 1967.*

Deane, H. W.: Some electron microscopic observations on the lamina propria of the gut, with comments on the close association of macrophages, plasma cells, and eosinophils. *Anat. Rec. 149:453, 1964.*

Dobbins, W. O., Herrero, B. A. and Mansbach, C. M.: Morphologic alterations associated with neomycin induced malabsorption. *Amer. J. Med. Sci. 255*:63, 1968.

Hampton, J. C.: Effects of fixation on the morphology of Paneth cell granules. *Stain Techn. 40*:283, 1965.

Hampton, J. C. and Rosario, B.: The passage of exogenous peroxidase from blood capillaries into the intestinal epithelium. *Anat. Rec. 159*:159, 1967.

Leeson, C. R. and Leeson, T. S.: The fine structure of Brunner's glands in the rabbit. *Anat. Rec. 159*:409, 1967.

Luse, S. A. and Lacy, P. E.: Electron microscopy of a malignant argentaffin tumor. *Cancer 13*:334, 1960.

Meader, R. D. and Landers, D. F.: Electron and light microscopic observations on relationships between lymphocytes and intestinal epithelium. *Amer. J. Anat. 121*:763, 1967.

Padykula, H. A., Strauss, E. W., Ladman, A. J. and Gardner, F. H.: A morphologic and histochemical analysis of the human jejunal epithelium in nontropical sprue. *Gastroenterology 40*:735, 1961.

Rostgaard, J. and Barrnett, R. J.: Fine structural observations of the absorption of lipid particles in the small intestine of the rat. *Anat. Rec. 152*:325, 1965.

Trier, J. S.: Structure of the mucosa of the small intestine as it relates to intestinal function. *Fed. Proc. 26*:1391, 1967.

Winborn, W. B.: Electron microscopic observations of dense bodies in parietal cells of the hamster. *Anat. Rec. 159*:387, 1967.

Large Intestine

Candiani, G. B., Lanzavecchia, G. and Mangioni, C.: Electron microscopic findings on the intestinal epithelium in rectal and sigmoid artificial bladders. *Exp. Molec. Path. 6*:402, 1967.

Hampton, J. C.: An electron microscopic study of mouse colon. *Dis. Colon Rectum 3*:423, 1960.

Schofield, G. C. and Silva, D. G.: The fine structure of enterochromaffin cells in the mouse colon. *J. Anat. 103*:1, 1968.

Silva, D. G., Farrell, K. E. and Smith, G. C.: Ultrastructural and histochemical studies on the innervation of the mucous membrane of the mouse colon. *Anat. Rec. 162*:157, 1968.

Venkatachaiam, M. A., Soltani, M. H. and Dariush Fahimi, H.: Fine structural localization of peroxidase activity in the epithelium of large intestine of rat. *J. Cell Biol. 46*:168, 1970.

Liver

Bronfenmajer, S., Schaffner, F. and Popper, H.: Fat-storage cells (lipocytes) in human liver. *Arch. Path. 82*:447, 1966.

Caramia, F., Ghergo, G. F. and Menghini, G.: A glycogen body in liver nuclei. *J. Ultrastruct. Res. 19*:573, 1967.

Chapman, G. B., Chiarodo, A. J., Coffey, R. J. and Wieneke, K.: The fine structure of mucosal epithelial cells of a pathological human gall bladder. *Anat. Rec. 154*:579, 1966.

DeMan, J. C. H. and Noorduyn, N. J. A.: Light and electron microscopic radioautography of hepatic cell nucleoli in mice treated with actinomycin D. *J. Cell Biol. 33*:489, 1967.

Dariush Fahimi, H.: The fine structural localization of endogenous and exogenous peroxidase activity in Kupffer cells of rat liver. *J. Cell Biol.* 47:247, 1970.

Elias, H. and Sherrick, J. C.: *Morphology of the Liver.* Academic Press, New York, 1969.

Fedorko, M. E., Hirsch, J. G. and Cohn, Z. A.: Autophagic vacuoles produced in vitro. 1. Studies on cultured macrophages exposed to chloroquine. *J. Cell Biol.* 38:377, 1968.

Fedorko, M. E., Hirsch, J. G. and Cohn, Z. A.: Autophagic vacuoles produced in vitro. 2. Studies on the mechanism of formation of autophagic vacuoles produced by chloroquine. *J. Cell Biol.* 38:392, 1968.

Goldfischer, S. and Bernstein, J.: Lipofuscin (aging) pigment granules of the newborn human liver. *J. Cell Biol.* 42:253, 1969.

Haust, M. D.: Crystalloid structures of hepatic mitochondria in children with heparitin sulphate mucopolysaccharidosis (Sanfilippo type). *Exp. Molec. Path.* 8:123, 1968.

Hollander, M. and Schaffner, F.: Electron microscopic studies in biliary atresia. 1. Bile ductular proliferation. *Amer. J. Dis. Child.* 116:49, 1968.

Hollander, M. and Schaffner, F.: Electron microscopic studies in biliary atresia. 2. Hepatocellular alterations. *Amer. J. Dis. Child.* 116:57, 1968.

Loud, A. V.: A quantitative stereological description of the ultrastructure of normal rat liver parenchymal cells. *J. Cell Biol.* 37:27, 1968.

Magalhães, M. M. and Magalhães, M. C.: Ultrastructural alterations produced in rat liver by metopiron. *J. Ultrastruct. Res.* 32:32, 1970.

Noorduyn, N. J. A. and DeMan, J. C.: RNA synthesis in rat and mouse hepatic cells as studied with light and electron microscopic radioautography. *J. Cell Biol.* 30:655, 1966.

Prose, P. H., Lee, L. and Balk, S. D.: Electron microscopic study of the phagocytic fibrin-clearing mechanism. *Amer. J. Path.* 47:403, 1965.

Rubin, E. and Lieber, C. S.: Experimental alcoholic hepatic injury in man: Ultrastructural changes. *Fed. Proc.* 26:1458, 1967.

Ruebner, B. H. and Slusser, R. J.: Hepatocytes and sinusoidal lining cells in viral hepatitis. *Arch. Path.* 86:1, 1968.

Ruffolo, R. and Covington, H.: Matrix inclusion bodies in the mitochondria of the human liver. *Amer. J. Path.* 51:101, 1967.

Satler, J.: Electron microscopy in the diagnostics of liver diseases. *Acta Hepatosplen.* 15:71, 1968.

Smith, J. R. C. and Reade, P. C.: An electron microscopical study of the uptake of foreign particles by the livers of foetal and adult rats. *Brit. J. Exp. Path.* 46:45, 1965.

Stein, O. and Stein, Y.: Lipid synthesis, intracellular transport, storage and secretion. 1. Electron microscopic radioautographic study of liver after injection of tritiated palmitate or glycerol in fasted and ethanol-treated rats. *J. Cell Biol.* 33:319, 1967.

Steiner, J. W., Phillips, M. J. and Miyai, K.: Ultrastructural and subcellular pathology of the liver. In *International Review of Experimental Pathology* (Richter, G. W. and Epstein, M. A., eds.). Academic Press, New York, 1964.

Sternlieb, I.: Perinuclear filaments and microtubules in human hepatocytes and biliary epithelial cells. *J. Microscopie* 4:551, 1965.

Trotter, N. L.: A fine structure of lipid in mouse liver regenerating after partial hepatectomy. *J. Cell Biol.* 21:233, 1964.

Wisse, E.: An electron microscopic study of the fenestrated endothelial lining of rat liver sinusoids. *J. Ultrastruct. Res.* 31:125, 1970.

Wood, R. L.: An electron microscopic study of developing bile canaliculi in the rat. *Anat. Rec. 151*:507, 1965.

Wood, R. L.: The fine structure of hepatic cells in chronic ethionine poisoning and during recovery. *Amer. J. Path. 46*:307, 1965.

Yamada, K.: Aspects of the fine structure of the intrahepatic bile duct epithelium in normal and cholecystectomized mice. *J. Morph. 124*:1, 1968.

Yamada, K.: Some observations on the fine structure of light and dark cells in the gall bladder epithelium of the mouse. *Z. Zellforsch. 84*:463, 1968.

Yamada, K.: Ultrastructural changes in liver parenchymal cells of the mouse following postnatal cholecystectomy. *Anat. Rec. 162*:373, 1968.

Zamboni, L.: Electron microscopic studies of blood embryogenesis in humans. 1. The ultrastructure of the fetal liver. *J. Ultrastruct. Res. 12*:509, 1965.

Zamboni, L.: Electron microscopic studies of blood embryogenesis in humans. 2. The hemopoietic activity in the fetal liver. *J. Ultrastruct. Res. 12*:525, 1965.

Exocrine Pancreas
Ciba Foundation on the Exocrine Pancreas. Little, Brown and Company, Boston, 1961.

Ekholm, R. and Edlund, Y.: Ultrastructure of the human exocrine pancreas. *J. Ultrastruct. Res. 2*:453, 1959.

Geuze, J. J.: Light and electron microscopic observations on auto- and heterophagy in the exocrine pancreas of the hibernating frog (Rana esculenta). *J. Ultrastruct. Res. 32*:391, 1970.

Kallman, F. and Grobstein, C.: Fine structure of differentiating mouse pancreatic exocrine cells in transfilter culture. *J. Cell Biol. 20*:399, 1964.

Lazarus, S. S. and Volk, B. W.: Electron microscopy and histochemistry of rabbit pancreas in protein malnutrition (experimental kwashiorkor). *Amer. J. Path. 44*:95, 1964.

Lazarus, S. S. and Volk, B. W.: Ultrastructure and acid phosphatase distribution in the pancreas of rabbits. *Arch. Path. 80*:135, 1965.

Legg, P. G.: Electron microscopic studies on compound tubular bodies in acinar cells of cat pancreas. *J. Anat. 103*:359, 1968.

Lever, J. D., Graham, J. D., Irvine, G. and Chick, W. J.: The vesiculated axons in relation to arteriolar smooth muscle in the pancreas. A fine structure and quantitative study. *J. Anat. 99*:299, 1965.

Lowe, H.: Elektronenmikroskopische studien zur proteinsynthese in der exokrinen pankreaszelle *in vivo* und *in vitro*. *Acta Biol. Med. German. 20*:655, 1968.

Martin, B. F., Levin, R. J. and Kugler, J. H.: A light and electron microscopic study of the exocrine pancreas following administration of 5-fluorouracil. *J. Anat. 104*:93, 1969.

Rosai, J.: Carcinoma of pancreas simulating giant cell tumor of bone. Electron-microscopic evidence of its acinar cell origin. *Cancer 22*:333, 1968.

Respiratory System

Ali, M. Y.: Histology of the human nasopharyngeal mucosa. *J. Anat. 99*:657, 1965.

Bargmann, W. and Knoop, A.: Vergleichende elektronenmikroskopische untersuchungen der lungenkapillaren. *Z Zellforsch. 44*:263, 1956.

Bensch, K. G., Gordon, G. B. and Miller, L. R.: Studies on the bronchial counterpart of the Kultschitzky (argentaffin) cell and innervation of bronchial glands. *J. Ultrastruct. Res. 12*:668, 1965.

Bertalanffy, F. D.: Respiratory tissue: Structure, histophysiology, cytodynamics. Parts 1–2. *Int. Rev. Cytol. 16*:233, 1964.

Bryan, W. T., Bryan, M. P. and Smith, C. A.: Cytochemical factors and some ultrastructural aspects of the epithelium in the secretions from nasal inflammatory diseases. *Laryngoscope 78*:1020, 1968.

Campiche, M.: Les inclusions lamellaires des cellules alveolaires dans le poumon du raton. Relations entre l'ultrastructure et la fixation. *J. Ultrastruct. Res. 3*:302, 1960.

Clemens, H. J.: Elektronenoptische untersuchungen über den bau der alveolenwand in der rattenlunge. *Z. Zellforsch. 40*:1, 1954.

Cottrell, T. S., Levine, O. R., Senior, R. M., Wiener, J., Spiro, D. and Fishman, A. P.: Electron microscopic alterations at the alveolar level in pulmonary edema. *Circ. Res. 21*:783, 1967.

Dalhamn, T.: Mucous flow and ciliary activity in the trachea of healthy rats and rats exposed to respiratory irritant gases. *Acta Physiol. Scand. 36*(Suppl.)123:1, 1956.

Dermer, G. B.: The pulmonary surfactant content of the inclusion bodies found within type II alveolar cells. *J. Ultrastruct. Res. 33*:306, 1970.

Dermer, G. B.: The fixation of pulmonary surfactant for electron microscopy. *J. Ultrastruct. Res. 31*:229, 1970.

Engström, H.: The structure of tracheal cilia. *Acta Otolaryng. 39*:360, 1951.

Frasca, J. M., Auerbach, O., Parks, V. R. and Stoeckenius, W.: Electron microscopic observations of bronchial epithelium. 1. Annulate lamellae. *Exp. Molec. Path. 6*:261, 1967.

Frasca, J. M., Auerbach, O., Parks, V. R. and Stoeckenius, W.: Electron microscopic observations of bronchial epithelium. 2. Filosomes. *Exp. Molec. Path. 7*:92, 1967.

Gieseking, R.: Elektronenoptische beobachtungen im alveolarbereich der lunge. *Beitr. Path. Anat. 116*:177, 1956.

Kalifat, S. R., Dupuy-Coin, A. M. and DeLarue, J.: Demonstration ultrastructurale de polysaccharides dont certain acides dan le film de surface de l'alveole pulmonaire. *J. Ultrastruct. Res. 32*:572, 1970.

Karrer, H. E.: The ultrastructure of mouse lung. A note on the fine structure of mitochondria and endoplasmic reticulum of the bronchiolar epithelium. *J. Biophys. Biochem. Cytol. 2*:115, 1956.

Karrer, H. E.: Electron microscopic study of bronchiolar epithelium of normal mouse lung. Preliminary report. *Exp. Cell Res. 10*:237, 1956.

Karrer, H. E.: The ultrastructure of mouse lung. The alveolar macrophage. *J. Biophys. Biochem. Cytol. 4*:693, 1958.

Klaus, M., Reiss, O. K., Tooley, W. H., Piel, C. and Clements, J. A.: Alveolar epithelial cell mitochondria as source of the surface-active lung lining. *Science 137*:750, 1962.

McNary, W. F. and El-Bermani, A.: Differentiating type I and type II alveolar cells in rat lung by O_sO4-NaI staining. *Stain Techn. 45*:215, 1970.

Policard, A., Collet, A. and Prégermain, S.: Le passage entre bronchioles et alvéoles pulmonaires. Étude au microscope électronique. *Presse Méd. 26*:999, 1960.

Urinary System

Glomerulus

Becker, E. L.: *Structural Basis of Renal Disease.* Hoeber Medical Division of Harper & Row, New York, 1968.

Benscome, S. A. and Bergman, B. J.: The ultrastructure of human and experimental glomerular lesions. In *International Review of Experimental Pathology*. (Richter, G. W. and Epstein, M. A., eds.). Academic Press, New York, 1962.

Blozis, G. G., Spargo, B. and Rowley, D. A.: Glomerular basement membrane changes with the nephrotic syndrome produced in the rat by homologous kidney and Hemophilus pertussis vaccine. *Amer. J. Path. 40*:153, 1962.

Cook, M. L., Osvaldo, L., Jackson, J. D. and Latta, H.: Changes in renal glomeruli during autolysis. Electron microscopic observations. *Lab. Invest. 14*:623, 1965.

Courtecuisse, V.: Aspect en microscopie electronique des lesions renales des micro-andiopathies a evolution curable. *Path. Biol. 15*:1087, 1967.

Dalton, A. J. and Haguenau, F.: *Ultrastructure of the Kidney*. Academic Press, New York, 1967.

De Martino, C. and Zamboni, L.: A morphologic study of the mesonephros of the human embryo. *J. Ultrastruct. Res. 16*:399, 1966.

Herdson, P. B., Jennings, R. B. and Earle, D. P.: Glomerular fine structure in poststreptococcal acute glomerulonephritis. *Arch. Path. 81*:117, 1966.

Jones, D. B., Mueller, C. B. and Menefee, M.: The cellular and extracellular morphology of the glomerular stalk. *Amer. J. Path. 41*:373, 1962.

Jorgensen, F.: Electron microscopic studies of normal visceral epithelial cells. *Lab. Invest. 17*:225, 1967.

Jorgensen, F. and Bentzon, M. W.: The ultrastructure of the normal human glomerulus; Thickness of glomerular basement membrane. *Lab. Invest. 18*:42, 1968.

Kimmelsteil, P.: Basement membrane in diabetic glomerulosclerosis. *Diabetes 15*:61, 1966.

Kimmelsteil, P., Osawa, G. and Beres, J.: Glomerular basement membranes in diabetics. *Amer. J. Clin. Path. 45*:21, 1966.

Latta, H.: The glomerular capillary wall. *J. Ultrastruct. Res. 32*:526, 1970.

Latta, H., Maunsbach, A. B. and Madden, S. C.: The centrolobular region of the renal glomerulus studied by electron microscopy. *J. Ultrastruct. Res. 4*:455, 1960.

Misra, R. P. and Berman, L. B.: Studies on glomerular basement membrane. 1. Isolation and chemical analysis of normal glomerular basement membrane. *Proc. Soc. Exp. Biol. Med. 122*:705, 1966.

Osawa, G., Kimmelsteil, P. and Seiling, V.: Thickness of glomerular basement membranes. *Amer. J. Clin. Path. 45*:7, 1966.

Suzuki, Y., Churg, J., Grishman, E., Mautner, W. and Dachs, S.: The mesangium of the renal glomerulus. Electron microscopic studies of pathologic alterations. *Amer. J. Path. 43*:555, 1963.

Tubules
Ericsson, J. L. E., Trump, B. F. and Weibel, J.: Electron microscopic studies of the proximal tubule of the rat kidney: 2. Cytosegresomes and cytosomes: Their relationship to each other and to the lysosome concept. *Lab. Invest. 14*:1341, 1965.

Ericsson, J. L. E., Andres, G., Bergstrand, A., Bucht, H. and Orsten, P. A.: Further studies on the fine structure of renal tubules in healthy humans. *Acta Path. Microbiol. Scand. 69*:493, 1967.

Latta, H., Osvaldo, L., Jackson, J. D. and Cook, M. L.: Changes in renal cortical tubules during autolysis. Electron microscopic observations. *Lab. Invest. 14*:635, 1965.

Olsen, T. S.: Ultrastructure of the renal tubules in acute renal insufficiency. *Acta Path. Microbiol. Scand.* 71:203, 1967.

Stone, R. S., Benscome, S. A., Latta, H. and Madden, S. C.: Renal tubular fine structure. Studied during reaction to acute uranium injury. *Arch. Path.* 71:160, 1961.

Stuve, J. and Galle, P.: Role of mitochondria in the handling of gold by the kidney. *J. Cell Biol.* 44:667, 1970.

Suzuki, T. and Mostofi, F. K.: Intramitochondrial filamentous bodies in the thick limb of Henle of the rat kidney. *J. Cell Biol.* 33:605, 1967.

Juxtaglomerular Apparatus

Barajas, L. and Latta, H.: Structure of the juxtaglomerular apparatus. *Circ. Res. Suppl.* 2, 20 & 21:11 & 15, 1967.

Barajas, L.: The ultrastructure of the juxtaglomerular apparatus as disclosed by three-dimensional reconstructions from serial sections. *J. Ultrastruct. Res.* 33:116, 1970.

Biava, C. and West, M.: Lipofuscin-like granules in vascular smooth muscle and juxtaglomerular cells of human kidneys. *Amer. J. Path.* 47:287, 1965.

Biava, C. G. and West, M.: Fine structure of normal human juxtaglomerular cells. 2. Specific and nonspecific cytoplasmic granules. *Amer. J. Path.* 49:955, 1966.

Biava, C. G.: Ultrastructural observations on the morphogenesis of nonspecific granules in human juxtaglomerular and renal vascular cells. *Circ. Res. Suppl. 2, 20 & 21:11 & 47,* 1967.

Fisher, E. R.: Lysosomal nature of juxtaglomerular granules. *Science* 152:1752, 1966.

Harada, K.: Rapid demonstration of juxtaglomerular granules with alcoholic crystal violet. *Stain Techn.* 45:71, 1970.

Hartroft, P. M.: The juxtaglomerular complex. *Bull. Path.* June:165, 1967.

Ureter and Urinary Bladder

DiBona, D. R. and Civan, M. M.: The effect of smooth muscle on the intracellular spaces in toad urinary bladder. *J. Cell Biol.* 46:235, 1970.

Monis, B. and Zambrano, D.: Transitional epithelium of urinary tract in normal and dehydrated rats. *Z. Zellforsch.* 85:165, 1968.

Special Sense—Eye and Ear

Eye

Allen, R. A.: Anatomy of the retina. *In Retinal Diseases* (Kimura, S. J. and Caygill, W. M., eds.). Lea and Febiger, Philadelphia, 1966.

Bairati, A., Jr., and Orzalesi, N.: The ultrastructure of the pigment epithelium and of the photoreceptor-pigment epithelium junction in the human retina. *J. Ultrastruct. Res.* 9:484, 1963.

Bernstein, M. H. and Hollenberg, M. J.: Fine structure of the choriocapillaris and retinal capillaries. In *Symposium on Vascular Disorders of the Eye. Basic Considerations in Anatomy and Physiology* (Bettman, J. W., ed.). C. V. Mosby Company, St. Louis, 1966.

Cohen, A. I.: New details of the ultrastructure of the outer segments and ciliary connectives of the rods of human and macaque retinas. *Anat. Rec.* 152:63, 1965.

Cohen, A. I.: Some electron microscopic observations on inter-receptor contacts in the human and macaque retinae. *J. Anat.* 99:595, 1965.

Jakus, M. A.: The fine structure of the human cornea. In *The Structure of the Eye* (Smelser, G. K., ed.). Academic Press, New York, 1961.

Magalhães, M. M. and Colmbra, A.: Electron microscope radioautographic study of glycogen synthesis in the rabbit retina. *J. Cell Biol. 47*:263, 1970.

Pedler, C. M. H. and Tilly, R.: The fine structure of photoreceptor discs. *Vision Res. 7*:829, 1967.

Stroke, G. W.: *An Introduction to Coherent Optics and Holography.* Academic Press, New York, 1969.

Tarkkanen, A. and Vannas, S.: Ultrastructure of Bruch's membrane in senile macular degeneration. *Acta Ophthal. 45*:694, 1967.

Tripathi, R. C.: Ultrastructure of Schlemm's canal in relation to aqueous outflow. *Exp. Eye Res. 7*:335, 1968.

Villegas, G. M.: Ultrastructure of the human retina. *J. Anat. 98*:501, 1964.

Yamamoto, T.: Sensory organ. In *Fine Structure of Cells and Tissues. Electron Microscopic Atlas* (Yamada, E., Yamamoto, T. and Hama, K., eds.). Igaku Shoin, Tokyo, 1968.

Yamashita, T. and Rosen, D. A.: Electron microscopic study of trabecular meshwork. In clinical and experimental glaucoma with anterior chamber hemorrhage. *Amer. J. Ophthal. 60*:427, 1965.

Young, R. W.: The renewal of photoreceptor cell outer segments. *J. Cell Biol. 33*:61, 1967.

Young, R. W.: Shedding of discs from rod outer segments in the Rhesus monkey. *J. Ultrastruct. Res. 34*:190, 1971.

Ear

Bredberg, G., Lindeman, H. H., Ades, H. W., and West, R.: Scanning electron microscopy of the organ of Corti. *Science 170*:861, 1970.

Duvall, A. J., Flock, A. and Wersall, J.: The ultrastructure of the sensory hairs and associated organelles of the cochlear inner hair cell, with reference to directional sensitivity. *J. Cell Biol. 29*:497, 1966.

Flock, A. and Duvall, A. J.: The ultrastructure of the kinocilium of the sensory cells in the inner ear and lateral line organs. *J. Cell Biol. 25*:1, 1965.

Johnson, F. R., McMinn, R. M. H. and Atfield, G. N.: Ultrastructural and biochemical observations on the tympanic membrane. *J. Anat. 103*:297, 1968.

Kawabata, I. and Paparella, M. M.: Ultrastructure of normal human middle ear mucosa. *Ann. Otol. 78*:125, 1969.

Yoshiaki, N. and Hilding, D. A.: Phosphotungstic acid staining of the organ of Corti by electron microscopy. *Anat. Rec. 162*:1, 1968.

Integumentary System

Epithelium

Breathnach, A. S. and Goodwin, D.: Electron microscopy of guinea-pig epidermis stained by the osmium-iodide technique. *J. Anat. 100*:159, 1966.

Breathnach, A. S. and Wyllie, L. M.: Fine structure of cells forming the surface layer of the epidermis in human fetuses at fourteen and twelve weeks. *J. Invest. Derm. 45*:179, 1965.

Brody, I.: Variations in the differentiation of the fibrils in the normal human stratum corneum as revealed by electron microscopy. *J. Ultrastruct. Res. 30*:601, 1970.

Brody, I.: An electron microscopic study of the fibrillar density in the normal human stratum corneum. *J. Ultrastruct. Res. 30:*209, 1970.

Cox, A. J. and Reaven, E. P.: Histidine and keratohyalin granules. *J. Invest. Derm. 49:*31, 1967.

Hoyes, A. D.: Electron microscopy of the surface layer (periderm) of human foetal skin. *J. Anat. 103:*321, 1968.

Matoltsy, A. G. and Matoltsy, M. N.: The chemical nature of keratohyalin granules of the epidermis. *J. Cell Biol. 47:*593, 1970.

Mustakallio, K. K. and Kiistala, U.: Electron microscopy of Merkel's "tastzelle," a potential monoamine storing cell of human epidermis. *Acta Dermatovener. 47:*323, 1967.

Nix, T. E., Nordquist, R. E. and Everett, M. A.: Ultrastructural changes induced by ultraviolet light in human epidermis: Granular and transitional cell layers. *J. Ultrastruct. Res. 12:*547, 1965.

Nix, T. E., Nordquist, R. E., Scott, J. R. and Everett, M. A.: Ultrastructural changes induced by ultraviolet light in human epidermis: Basal and spinous layers. *J. Invest. Derm. 45:*52, 1965.

Odland, G. F.: The fine structure of the interrelationship of cells in the human epidermis. *J. Biophys. Biochem. Cytol. 4:*529, 1958.

Odland, G. F.: A submicroscopic granular component in human epidermis. *J. Invest. Derm. 34:*11, 1960.

Prose, P. H., Kien, A. E. F. and Neistein, S.: Ultrastructural studies of organ cultures of adult human skin. In vitro growth and keratinization of epidermal cells. *Lab. Invest. 17:*693, 1967.

Ross, R. and Odland, G.: Human wound repair. I. Epidermal regeneration. *J. Cell Biol. 39:*135, 1968.

Ross, R. and Odland, G.: Human wound repair. II. Inflammatory cells, epithelial-mesenchymal interrelations, and fibrogenesis. *J. Cell Biol. 39:*152, 1968.

Snell, R.: An electron microscopic study of the human epidermal keratinocyte. *Z. Zellforsch. 79:*492, 1967.

Zelickson, A. S. (ed.): *Electron Microscopy of Skin and Mucous Membrane.* Charles C Thomas, Springfield, 1963.

Zelickson, A. S. (ed.): *Ultrastructure of Normal and Abnormal Skin.* Lea and Febiger, Philadelphia, 1967.

Hair

Breathnach, A. S. and Smith, J.: Fine structure of the early hair germ and dermal papilla in the human foetus. *J. Anat. 102:*511, 1968.

Nakai, T.: A study of the ultrastructural localization of hair keratin synthesis utilizing electron microscopic autoradiography in a magnetic field. *J. Cell Biol. 21:*63, 1964.

Glands

Biempica, L. and Montes, L. F.: Secretory epithelium of the large axillary sweat glands. A cytochemical and electron microscopic study. *Amer. J. Anat. 117:*47, 1965.

Hashimoto, K., Gross, B. G. and Lever, W. F.: The ultrastructure of the skin of human embryos. 1. The intraepidermal eccrine sweat duct. *J. Invest. Derm. 45:*139, 1965.

Munger, B. L.: The cytology of apocrine sweat glands. 2. Human. *Z. Zellforsch. 68:*837, 1965.

Pigment

Breathnach, A. S., Fitzpatrick, T. B. and Wyllie, L. M. A.: Electron microscopy of melanocytes in human piebaldism. *J. Invest. Derm. 45:28*, 1965.

Mottaz, J. H. and Zelickson, A. S.: Melanin transfer: A possible phagocytic process. *J. Invest. Derm. 49:605*, 1967.

Zelickson, A. S. (ed.): *Ultrastructure of Normal and Abnormal Skin*. Lea and Febiger, Philadelphia, 1967.

Tooth

Garant, P. R.: An electron microscopic study of the crystal-matrix relationship in the teeth of dogfish Squalus acanthias L. *J. Ultrastruct. Res. 30:441*, 1970.

Kallenbach, E.: Fine structure of rat incisor enamel organ during late pigmentation and regression stages. *J. Ultrastruct. Res. 30:38*, 1970.

Lester, K. S.: On the nature of "fibrils" and tubules in developing enamel of the opossum, Didelphis marsupialis. *J. Ultrastruct. Res. 30:64*, 1970.

Lester, K. S. and Boyde, A.: Scanning electron microscopy of developing roots of molar teeth of the laboratory rat. *J. Ultrastruct. Res. 33:80*, 1970.

Listgarten, M. A.: A light and electron microscopic study of coronal cementogenesis. *Arch. Oral Biol. 13:93*, 1968.

Provenza, D. V., Fischlschweiger, W. and Sisca, R. F.: Fibres in human dental papillae. A preliminary report on the fine structure. *Arch. Oral Biol. 12:1533*, 1967.

Reith, E. J.: The stages of amelogenesis as observed in molar teeth of young rats. *J. Ultrastruct. Res. 30:111*, 1970.

Searls, J. C.: Light and electron microscope evaluation of changes induced in odontoblasts of the rat incisor by the high-speed drill. *J. Dent. Res. 46:1344*, 1967.

Selvig, K. A.: Ultrastructural changes in human dentine exposed to weak acid. *Arch. Oral Biol. 13:719*, 1968.

INDEX

All figures refer to *plate numbers*. Plate numbers in *italics* indicate primary descriptions of structures.

Bruch's membrane, 142
Brunner's glands, 110
Brush border, 133
Bud(s), taste, 105

C CAJAL'S GOLD CHLORIDE METHOD, 63
Calcification, 29, 30, 150
Calcium
   in bone, 30
   in dentin, 150
   in muscle, 48, 49, 98
Calyces of kidneys, 135
Canal(s)
   haversian, 32
   of Schlemm, 138
   of Volkmann, 32
Canaliculi
   bile, 10, 115, *116*, 118
   of bone, 31, 32
   intracellular, *107*, 108
Cancellous bone, 31, 32
Capillary(ies), 14, 54, 55, *69*, 74, 75, 76, 77, 78, 80, 81,
     83, 101, 102, 125, 126, 129, 130, 131, 132
Capsule(s)
   of adrenal gland, 80
   Bowman's, *130*, 133
   of cartilage cell, 35
   of ganglion, 60
   of kidney, 130
   of lens, 140
   of lymph nodes, 70
   of spleen, 71
   of testis, 85
   of thymus, 72
Carbon, 24, 129
Cardiac muscle, 12, *54*, 55
Cartilage
   cells of, 29, 34
   elastic, *34*, 124
   fibro-, *35*
   hyaline, 29, 35, 123, 127
Carotenoid(s), 83
Catalase, 115
Catecholamine(s), 81
Cell(s)
   A cells of testis, 85
   A cells of pancreas, 84
   acidophil, of pituitary, 75, 76
   adipose, 9, *25*
   alveolar, 126
   anterior horn, of spinal cord, 58
   argentaffin, 109, 110, 113, *114*
   astrocytes, 59, 63
   B cells of pancreas, 84
   B cells of pituitary, 75
   B cells of testis, 85
   basal, of epidermis, 146
   basophil, of pituitary, 75, 76
   Betz, 59
   bipolar, 142, 143, 144

Cell(s) (*Continued*)
   blood, 36, 37, 38, 39, 40, 41, 42, 43, 44, 45, 70, 71,
     72, 74
   cardiac muscle, 54, 55
   cartilage, 29, 34
   centroacinar, 121
   chief
     of parathyroid, 79
     of stomach, 5, 107, 108
   chromphil, of pituitary, 75, 76
   chromophobe, of pituitary, 75, 76
   Clara, 127
   clasmatocyte, 128
   decidual, 97, 101
   Deiter's, 144, 145
   dust, 128
   endothelial, 14, 36, 63, 64, 66, 67, 68, 69, 72, 73,
     78, 125, 126, 129, 130, 131, 132, 141
   enterochromaffin (argentaffin), 109, 110, 113, 114
   epithelial, 14, 15, 16, 17, 18, 19, 20
   fat, 9, 25
   fibroblast, *22*, 23, 26, *47*, 56, 57, 68, 74, 86, 89, 90,
     97, 99, 100, 126
   follicular, of ovary, 83, 92, 93, 95
   ganglion, 60, 81, 142, 143
   glial, 58, 63, 64
   glomerular epithelial (podocytes), 14, 130, 131,
     132
   goblet, *17*, 110, *111*, 113, 114, 122, 123, 127
   gonadotroph of pituitary, 75
   granulosa, 92, 93, 95
   hair, of organ of Corti, 144, 145
   hepatic, 10, 115, 116, 117, 118
   interstitial (Leydig), of testis, *82*, 85
   Kupffer, 3, 115, 116, *117*
   luteal, 83
   macrophage, 3, *24*, 117, 128
   mast, *26*
   megakaryocyte, 45, *46*
   melanocyte, 12, *28*
   mesangial, 131
   mesenchymal, 21, 97
   monocyte, 4, *42*
   mucous, 4, 16, 21, 103, 107, 108, 109, 110
   Muller, 142
   myeloblast, 37, *39*, 46
   myocardial, 12, *54*, 55
   myoepithelial (basket), 103, 104
   neuron, 56, 57, 58, 59, 60, 61, 62, 142, 143
   neuroepithelial, of taste, 105
   neuroglial, 59, 61, 62, *63*, 64
   neurosecretory, 75
   odontoblast, 150
   oligodendroglia, 64
   oocyte, 92, 93, 94, 95
   osteoblast, 31
   osteoclast, 33
   osteocyte, 32
   oxyphil, of parathyroid gland, 79
   Paneth, 110, 112

374

Marrow, 37, 39, 46
Mast cells, *26*
Matrix
  of bone, 31, 32, 33
  of cartilage, 29, 30, 124
Media of blood vessels, 66, 67, 68
Mediastinum testis, 85
Medulla(e)
  of adrenal gland, 81
  of kidney, 130, *135*
  of lymph node, 70
  of thymus, 72, 73
Medullary cavity of bone, 31
Medullary ray, 130, 133, *135*
Megakaryocyte(s), 45, *46*
Meiosis, 85, 92
Meissner's corpuscle(s), 65
Melanin pigment, 12, 28, 141, 142, 143
Melanocyte(s), 12, 141
Membrane(s)
  of Bowman, 138
  Bruch's, 142
  of Descemet, 138, 139
  limiting, 142
  mucous, 122
  Reissner's vestibular, 144
Menstrual cycle, 97, 98
Mesangial cell(s), 131
Mesaxon, 56, 57
Mesenchymal cell(s), *21*, 97
Mesothelial cell(s), 14
Metacentric position of centromere, 13
Metachromasia, 26, 41
Metamyelocyte(s), 38, *39*
Metaphase, 13, 29
Methylene azure, 38
Microbody(ies), 5, 77, 78, 115, 117
Microfilament(s), 45
Microtubule(s), 45, 56, 58, 61, 64, 144
Microvilli, 3, 15, 16, 17, 69, 77, 78, 88, 89, 90, 91, 93,
    96, 97, 99, 100, 101, 102, 105, 110, *111*, 112,
    115, 116, 119, 120, 121, 126, 128, 129, 133, 134,
    136
Midbody of spermatozoan, 87
Mitochondria, 1, *2*, 24, 32, 33, 37, 43, 44, 45, 46, 51,
    77, 78, 79, 80, 83, 84, 86, 92, 104, 115, 117,
    119, 123, 129, 134
  granules of, 2, 32, 98
Mitosis, 13
Modiolus, 144
Molecular layer of cerebral cortex, 61
Monocyte(s), 4, *42*
Motor neurons, 58
Mucoid ground substance, 21
Mucopolysaccharide(s), 29
Mucosa, 106, 113, 123, 136, 137
Mucous cell(s), 4, 16, 21, 103, 107, 108, 109, 110
Mucous gland(s), 106, 109, 110, 122, 123
Mucus, 4, 111
Muller cell(s), 142
Multipolar cell(s), 58, 59, 61

Multivesicular body(ies), 24, 93
Muscle(s)
  cardiac, 12, *54, 55*
  skeletal, *47, 48*, 49, 50, 51
  smooth, *52, 53*, 66, 67, 68, 88, 89, 90, 91, 98, 113,
    136, 137, 141
  voluntary, *47, 48*, 49, 50, 51
Muscular arteries, 66
Muscularis externa, 106
Muscularis mucosa, 106
Myelin figure(s), 3, *9*, 117
Myelin sheath(s), *56, 57*, 58, 59, 64
Myeloblast(s), 37, *39*, 46
Myelocyte(s), 38, *39*
Myocardial cell(s), 12, *54, 55*
Myoepithelial (basket) cell(s), 103, 104
Myofibril(s), 48, *49, 50*, 54, 55
Myofilament(s), *47, 48, 49, 50*, 51, 52, 53, 54, 55, 68,
    98, 141
Myometrium, *97*, 98
Myosin, 47, 48, *49, 50*, 51, 52, 53, 54, 55

NASAL EPITHELIUM, 122
Neck of gastric glands, 107, 108
Nephron(s), 14, 130, 131, 132, 133, 134, 135
Nerve(s)
  auditory, 144, 145
  autonomic, 60
  endings of, 51, 65
  fibers of, 56, 57
  myelinated, 56, 57
  nonmyelinated, 56, 57
  optic, 142
  parasympathetic, 137
  peripheral, 56, 57
Nervous system, 56, 57, 58, 59, 60, 61, 62, 63, 64, 65
Neurectoderm, 81
Neurilemma, 56, 57
Neuroepithelial cell(s) of taste, 105
Neurofibril(s), 56, 57, 58, 61, 63, 64
Neurohypophysis, 75
Neuroglial cell(s), 59, 61, *63*, 64
Neuromuscular junction(s), 51
Neuron(s), 56, 57, 58, 59, 60, 61, 62, 142, 143
Neuropil(s), 59
Neurosecretory cell(s), 75
Neutrophil granulocyte(s), 3, 7, 38
Nissl body(ies), *58*, 60
Node(s) of Ranvier, 56
Nodule(s), lymph, 44, 69, 70, 71, 74, 112, 114
Norepinephrine, 81
Normoblast(s), 37
Nuclear membrane(s), 6
Nuclear pore(s), *1*, 6, 92, 93, 94, 137
Nucleolonema, *6*
Nucleolus, *6*
Nucleus, *7*, 27, 37, 38, 46, 92, 99, 115, 119, 120, 123,
    131, 132, 137

ODONTOBLAST(S), 150
Oligodendrocyte(s), 64

N

O

DATE DUE

JAN 24 73			
OCT 30 '73			
FEB 12 '74			
JAN 25 '77			
MAY 9 '78			
MAR 20 '79			
AUG 17 '82			
FEB 15 '88			
JUN 14 '83			
OCT 3 '87			

GAYLORD   PRINTED IN U.S.A.